LABORATORY MATHEMATICS

medical and biological applications

LABORATORY MATHEMATICS

medical and biological applications

JUNE BLANKENSHIP, M.Ed., M.T. (ASCP)
JOE BILL CAMPBELL, Ph.D.

with 39 illustrations

THE C. V. MOSBY COMPANY

Saint Louis   *1976*

Library of Congress Cataloging in Publication Data

Blankenship, June, 1933-
    Laboratory mathematics: medical and biological applications.

    Bibliography: p.
    Includes index.
    1. Medicine, Clinical. 2. Medicine—Mathematics.
I. Campbell, Joe Bill, 1941-   joint author.
II. Title. [DNLM: 1. Mathematics. 2. Technology,
Medical. 3. Diagnosis, Laboratory. QA37 B642L]
RB38.2.B55   616.07'5'0151   75-15598
ISBN 0-8016-0700-0

GW/M/M   9 8 7 6 5 4 3 2

Preface

Mathematics is a science, a set of concepts, a way of thinking, a tool, and a mystery. It is all of these things to everyone. However, the importance of each property varies with different people. To the people who work in laboratories, the two most significant are its function as a tool and its tendency to remain a mystery.

Often the education and training of laboratory personnel is incomplete in the manipulation of values. The most painful aspect of this deficiency is that the laboratory worker cannot find a reference book through which needed knowledge can be gained. This book is offered to help such personnel. It provides simplified explanations of the calculations commonly used in the clinical and general biological laboratory.

This book is a beginning, not an end. It has been written to help the student with an inadequate background in math develop essential mastery needed for clinical performance. It also will be a useful refresher for the laboratory worker who needs strengthening in specific areas.

We have attempted to present the explanations in such a manner that the reader can understand each step of the calculation. Also a brief explanation of the chemical and physical principles involved with the calculation is given. The explanations presented here are meant to show how to do the problems, with enough theory to continue study. This text is not considered to be a complete book on the theory of mathematics.

We fully recognize the existence of imperfections in this work and will gratefully accept any criticisms and suggestions that may improve this book. We hope that it will prove to be a useful aid for those who do the actual laboratory work.

June Blankenship
Joe Bill Campbell

Contents

LABORATORY MATHEMATICS

medical and biological applications

CHAPTER 1

Basic mathematics

GENERAL CONCEPTS

Students of laboratory technology have a varying degree of expertise in mathematics. This chapter considers some basic concepts of mathematics that anyone completing 12 years of public education should know. However, we realize that in many schools the goal is not that of disseminating useful knowledge but of sheltering incompetent personnel and frustrating competent teachers. This book cannot cover every aspect of mathematics and still remain within its designed scope. This chapter provides a review of the major concepts of mathematics needed for the technical aspects of most medical and biological laboratories. If the student does not understand these concepts after studying the review in this chapter, further sources of study should be sought to learn enough about the science and application of mathematics to use this book.

In so far as possible, the student should not only understand how to do mathematical calculations but should understand why the manipulations of the figures work as they do. When a formula is presented as a method of solution to a problem, the student should attempt to understand the principle on which the formula is based. Understanding the basis of a formula often allows one to modify the formula to better suit a particular situation.

In doing mathematical calculations there are several general considerations to make in order to determine the most efficient method of solving the problem and to reduce error. Some of these are as follows:

1. Read the problem carefully. Be sure the entire problem has been read and understood.
2. Determine what principles and relationships are involved.
3. Determine exactly what results are to be produced by the calculations.
4. Think about the possible methods to use in solving the problem.
5. Write the intermediate stages of the calculations clearly. Avoid writing one number on top of another as a method of correction. Make each digit legible.
6. Recognize different forms of the same value, such as: $^1/_2$, 1/2, $1 \div 2$, 0.5, 50%, and 0.50.
7. Be extremely careful in positioning the decimal point.
8. Mentally estimate an answer before working the problem; compare the calculated result with the estimated answer. If the two figures disagree drastically, determine which is wrong.

MANIPULATION OF SIGNED NUMBERS

The "+" and "−" have two uses in mathematics. One use is to indicate the addition and subtraction operations. The other use is to determine the direction of progression of a number from zero. Numbers are used to denote a progression of values from a beginning point. The beginning point is zero. A concept of numbers that is overlooked by many people is that the progression of values moves away from zero in two directions.

$$\longleftarrow \text{Infinity} \quad -7 \quad -6 \quad -5 \quad -4 \quad -3 \quad -2 \quad -1 \quad 0 \quad +1 \quad +2 \quad +3 \quad +4 \quad +5 \quad +6 \quad +7 \quad \text{Infinity} \longrightarrow$$

Customarily numbers to the right of the zero point are spoken of as *positive numbers*, whereas numbers to the left of zero are spoken of as *negative numbers*.

1. Addition of positive and negative numbers.

   a. Addition of positive numbers: add all numbers and give the sum a positive sign.

$$\begin{array}{r} (+)4 \\ +(+)2 \\ \hline (+)6 \end{array}$$

   b. Addition of negative numbers: add all numbers and give the sum a negative sign.

$$\begin{array}{r} (-)4 \\ +(-)2 \\ \hline (-)6 \end{array}$$

   c. Addition of positive and negative numbers: add the following numbers.

$$\begin{array}{r} (+)6 \\ (-)3 \\ (-)2 \\ +(+)1 \end{array}$$

First, add all the positive numbers.

$$\begin{array}{r} (+)6 \\ +(+)1 \\ \hline (+)7 \end{array}$$

Second, add all the negative numbers.

$$\begin{array}{r} (-)3 \\ +(-)2 \\ \hline (-)5 \end{array}$$

Subtract the smaller sum from the larger sum and give the answer the sign of the larger sum.

$$\begin{array}{r} (+)7 \\ +(-)5 \\ \hline (+)2 \end{array}$$

2. Subtraction with positive and negative numbers. To subtract, replace the sign of the number being subtracted with its opposite and then add.

   a. Subtraction of positive numbers (see c under addition)

$$\begin{array}{r} (+)4 \\ -(+)2 \\ \hline \end{array} \qquad \begin{array}{r} (+)4 \\ +(-)2 \\ \hline (+)2 \end{array}$$

   b. Subtraction of a negative number from a positive number (see a under addition)

$$\begin{array}{r} (+)4 \\ -(-)2 \\ \hline \end{array} \qquad \begin{array}{r} (+)4 \\ +(+)2 \\ \hline (+)6 \end{array}$$

   c. Subtraction of a greater positive number from a lesser positive number (see c under addition)

$$\begin{array}{cc} (+)42 & (+)42 \\ \underline{-(+)72} & \underline{+(-)72} \end{array} \qquad \begin{array}{c} (-)72 \\ \underline{+(+)42} \\ (-)30 \end{array}$$

d. Subtraction of a positive number from a negative number (see b under addition)

$$\begin{array}{cc} (-)4 & (-)4 \\ \underline{-(+)3} & \underline{+(-)3} \\ & (-)7 \end{array}$$

3. Multiplication of positive and negative numbers.
    a. A positive number × a positive number = a positive number

$$+4 \times +4 = +16$$

   b. A positive number × a negative number = a negative number

$$+4 \times -4 = -16$$

   c. A negative number × a positive number = a negative number

$$-4 \times +4 = -16$$

   d. A negative number × a negative number = a positive number

$$-4 \times -4 = +16$$

4. Division of positive and negative numbers.
    a. A positive number ÷ a positive number = a positive number

$$+20 \div +5 = +4$$

   b. A positive number ÷ a negative number = a negative number

$$+20 \div -5 = -4$$

   c. A negative number ÷ a positive number = a negative number

$$-20 \div +5 = -4$$

   d. A negative number ÷ a negative number = a positive number

$$-20 \div -5 = +4$$

ORDER OF CALCULATIONS

Sometimes in a problem it may be necessary to carry out several types of computations. There is an established *order* in which these operations should be carried out.
1. Order of operations when there are no parentheses: multiply and divide from left to right; then, add and subtract.

$$3 \times 4 + 6 - 8 \div 2 + 1 \times 4$$

Multiply and divide first from left to right.

$$(3 \times 4) + 6 - (8 \div 2) + (1 \times 4)$$
$$12 + 6 - 4 + 4$$
$$22 - 4 = 18$$

2. Order of operations within parentheses: do operations within the parentheses first; then, treat the result as one number in the operation.

$$(3 + 6 - 2) + (4 \times 2 + 1) - (6 - 4 \div 2)$$
$$(7) + [(4 \times 2) + 1] - [6 - (4 \div 2)]$$

$$(7) + (8 + 1) - (6 - 2)$$
$$(7) + (9) - (4)$$
$$7 + 9 - 4$$
$$16 - 4 = 12$$

3. Order of operations for groupings within a grouping: simplify the innermost grouping first and work outward; then proceed as in 1.

$$\{9 - [7 + (4 \div 2) - 1]\}$$
$$[9 - (7 + 2 - 1)]$$
$$9 - 8 = 1$$

COMMON FRACTIONS

The word *fraction* comes from the same Latin root as *fragment,* signifying a part. In expressing fractional division, it should be understood that all of the parts into which the object has been divided are of equal size. A common fraction consists of two parts: (1) an upper number, the numerator, which signifies the number of total parts present, and (2) a lower number, the denominator, which signifies the total number of divisions.

Any fraction in which the numerator is smaller than the denominator is called a *proper* fraction. Any fraction in which the numerator is larger than the denominator is called an *improper* fraction.

An improper fraction may be written as an integer followed by a fraction; this is called a *mixed number*.

1. Addition of fractions. In the addition of fractions the denominators must be the same. If the denominators are alike, add the numerators and place the sum over the denominator.

$$\frac{3}{7} + \frac{6}{7} = \frac{9}{7}$$

If the denominators are not alike, convert them to like terms; then, proceed as above.

$$\frac{1}{2} + \frac{1}{3} = \frac{3}{6} + \frac{2}{6} = \frac{5}{6}$$

2. Subtraction of fractions. In the subtraction of fractions the denominators must all be the same. If the denominators are alike, subtract the numerators in the indicated manner and place the difference over the denominator.

$$\frac{4}{6} - \frac{1}{6} = \frac{3}{6}$$

If the denominators are not alike, convert them to like terms; then, proceed as above.

$$\frac{5}{7} - \frac{1}{3} = \frac{15}{21} - \frac{7}{21} = \frac{8}{21}$$

3. Multiplication of fractions. To multiply one fraction by another, multiply the numerators of the fractions times each other and multiply the denominators of the fractions times each other.

$$\frac{1}{3} \times \frac{2}{5} = \frac{2}{15}$$

When mixed numbers are to be multiplied, change each mixed number to an improper fraction and proceed as above.

$$1\frac{1}{5} \times 2\frac{2}{6} = \frac{6}{5} \times \frac{14}{6} = \frac{84}{30} = \frac{14}{5} = 2\frac{4}{5}$$

4. Division of fractions. To divide one fraction by another, invert the fraction being divided (by making the numerator the denominator and vice versa) and multiply.

$$\frac{3}{6} \div \frac{4}{5} = \frac{3}{6} \times \frac{5}{4} = \frac{15}{24}$$

To divide mixed numbers, convert them to improper fractions and proceed as above.

DECIMAL FRACTIONS

Another method used to express a part of a whole number is by use of the decimal fraction or simply decimal. The decimal is actually the number of parts of one. The decimal fraction is indicated by the decimal point. Any common fraction can be expressed as a decimal fraction by dividing the numerator by the denominator.

$$\frac{1}{2} = 0.5$$

Often a common fraction cannot be converted into a decimal exactly. In such cases these numbers should be rounded off according to rules discussed later in this chapter.

$$\frac{1}{3} = 0.333333333 = 0.33 = 0.3$$

$$\frac{2}{3} = 0.666666666 = 0.67 = 0.7$$

1. Addition or subtraction of numbers containing decimals. Align the decimal point of each number, one directly under the other and add or subtract as discussed earlier. The decimal point of the answer will remain aligned with the points of the numbers of the problem.

$$\begin{array}{r} 0.62 \\ 0.103 \\ +0.01 \\ \hline 0.733 \end{array} \qquad \begin{array}{r} 0.762 \\ -0.15 \\ \hline 0.612 \end{array}$$

2. Multiplication of numbers containing decimal fractions. The number of digits to the right of the decimal point of the answer equals the total number of digits to the right of the decimal points of the numbers involved in the calculation.

$$\begin{array}{r} 7.43 \\ \times 3.45 \\ \hline 3715 \\ 2972 \\ 2229 \\ \hline 25.6335 \end{array}$$

3. Division of one decimal number by another. Arrange the numbers as if whole numbers were being divided.

$$6.78\overline{)74.934}$$

Move the decimal point of the divisor (the number by which division is being made) to the right of the last digit. Move the decimal point of the dividend (the number being divided) to the right a number of spaces equal to the number of spaces the decimal point of the divisor was moved.

$$6.\underset{\curvearrowright}{78.}\,\overline{)74.\underset{\curvearrowright}{93.}4}$$

Place the decimal point of the answer directly above the new position of the decimal point of the dividend.

$$678\overline{)7493.\overset{\cdot}{4}}$$

Complete the calculations.

$$
\begin{array}{r}
11.05 \\
678\overline{)7493.4} \\
\underline{678} \\
713 \\
\underline{678} \\
3540 \\
\underline{3390} \\
150
\end{array}
$$

The number of decimal places can be increased by placing a zero after the remainder and continuing the division process.

EQUATIONS

The equal sign "=" is much used in mathematics and means that the result of all material on one side of this sign must equal the result of all material on the other side. This is one of the basic principles of the part of mathematics called *algebra,* and the expression is called an *equation.* Problems are set up using all the known values, and a letter, usually *X,* is substituted for the unknown value. The equal sign divides the setup in such a manner as to produce two equal parts if the unknown values become known.

$$
\begin{aligned}
X &= 2 + 3 \\
X &= 5 \\
5 &= 5
\end{aligned}
$$

The calculated value on one side of an equation must be the same as the calculated value on the other side. The following are some general rules to use in calculating problems set up as equations:

1. Both sides of the equation must produce the same value when solved.

$$
\begin{aligned}
X &= 2 + 3 \\
X &= 5 \\
5 &= 5
\end{aligned}
$$

2. Generally, it is easier to solve a problem if all known material is moved to one side of the equation and all unknown material is moved to the other side.

3. When a part to be added or subtracted in an equation is moved to the other side of the equal sign, the sign of the part being moved is changed.

$$
\begin{aligned}
4 + X &= 2 + 3 \\
X &= 2 + 3 - 4 \\
X &= 5 - 4 \\
X &= 1
\end{aligned}
\qquad\qquad
\begin{aligned}
X - 7 &= 17 \\
X &= 17 + 7 \\
X &= 24
\end{aligned}
$$

Proof:

$$
\begin{aligned}
4 + 1 &= 2 + 3 \\
5 &= 5
\end{aligned}
\qquad\qquad
\begin{aligned}
24 - 7 &= 17 \\
17 &= 17
\end{aligned}
$$

4. When numbers of an equation are to be multiplied or divided, they can be more easily handled if expressed as common fractions.

$$X \div 7 = 9 \times 3 \div 4$$

$$\frac{X}{7} = \frac{9 \times 3}{4}$$

When such fractional expressions are moved from one side of an equation to the other, they are inverted.

$$\frac{X}{7} = \frac{9 \times 3}{4}$$

$$X = \frac{9 \times 3}{4} \times \frac{7}{1}$$

$$X = \frac{189}{4}$$

$$X = 47.25$$

If both sides of an equation are turned over, the equality remains the same.

$$\frac{7}{X} = \frac{4}{27} \qquad\qquad \frac{X}{7} = \frac{27}{4}$$

$$4X = 7 \times 27 \qquad\qquad 4X = 27 \times 7$$

$$X = \frac{7 \times 27}{4} \qquad\qquad X = \frac{27 \times 7}{4}$$

$$X = \frac{189}{4} \qquad\qquad X = \frac{189}{4}$$

$$X = 47.25 \qquad\qquad X = 47.25$$

RECIPROCALS

A reciprocal is the multiplicative inverse of a number. The product of a number and its reciprocal is always equal to one. A number and its reciprocal have the same sign.

The reciprocal of 2 is $^1/_2$ or 0.5.

$$2 \times \frac{1}{2} = \frac{2}{2} = 1$$

$$0.5 \times 2 = 1$$

The reciprocal of 8 is $^1/_8$ or 0.125.

$$\frac{8}{1} \times \frac{1}{8} = \frac{8}{8} = 1$$

$$8 \times 0.125 = 1$$

The reciprocal of -7 is $-^1/_7$.

$$-\frac{7}{1} \times -\frac{1}{7} = +\frac{7}{7} = +1$$

The reciprocal of $^2/_3$ is $^3/_2$.

$$\frac{2}{3} \times \frac{3}{2} = \frac{6}{6} = 1$$

EXPONENTS

Exponents are used to indicate that a number is to be multiplied by itself. The number to be multiplied by itself is called the *base*. The small superior numbers indicate how many times the number is to be used in the multiplication.

$$10^2 = 10 \times 10 = 100$$
$$10^4 = 10 \times 10 \times 10 \times 10 = 10,000$$
$$6^3 = 6 \times 6 \times 6 = 216$$

Negative exponents are used to represent the multiplication of fractions; or, stated another way, the reciprocal of the number is to be used.

$$10^{-1} = 1/10 = 0.1$$
$$10^{-3} = 1/10 \times 1/10 \times 1/10 = 1/1000 = 0.001$$
$$2^{-3} = 1/2 \times 1/2 \times 1/2 = 1/8$$

Rules of exponents

Letters are sometimes used to indicate numbers. This is especially useful in stating general rules. The letters m and n have been used to represent integers in the following rules of exponents:

1. To multiply two numbers *having the same base,* write the base with the exponents added.

$$a^m \times a^n = a^{m + n}$$
$$6^2 \times 6^3 = 6^{2 + 3} = 6^5$$

2. To raise an exponential number to a higher power, multiply the two exponents.

$$(a^m)^n = a^{mn}$$
$$(6^2)^3 = 6^{2 \times 3} = 6^6$$

3. To divide one number by another number *having the same base,* write the base with the exponents subtracted.

$$\frac{a^m}{a^n} = a^{m - n}$$

$$\frac{6^3}{6^2} = 6^{3 - 2} = 6^1 = 6$$

To multiply or divide numbers having different bases, it is necessary to convert the exponent numbers to the corresponding simple numbers. Then, complete the calculations using these numbers.

EXAMPLE: $2^3 \times 10^2$

$$2^3 = 2 \times 2 \times 2 = 8$$
$$10^2 = 10 \times 10 = 100$$

$$8 \times 100 = 800$$

SIGNIFICANT FIGURES

A number is an expression of quantity. The terms *figure* and *digit* are applied to any of the characters 0 and 1 to 9, which are used, either alone or in combination, to express numbers.

A significant figure may be defined as a digit that denotes the amount of the quantity in the spot in which it stands. Stated another way, a significant figure is one that is known to be reasonably reliable.

Since in all chemical determinations the accuracy is limited by all the steps involved (such as human error, pipetting, reagent reliability, and instrument accuracy), the reported result should give some indication of the reliability of the measurement by the number of significant figures that are in that result. For example, if the result of a test

Table 1

Result	Number of significant figures	Implied limit
10	2	9.5 to 10.5
10.5	3	10.45 to 10.55
10.50	4	10.495 to 10.505

was reported as 10.5, this should mean that the result was accurate to the nearest tenth and that the exact value was between 10.45 and 10.55. If this result had been reliable to the nearest hundredth, it would have been reported as 10.50. The number of significant figures is different in each example. The figure 10.5 contains three significant figures, but 10.50 contains four significant figures. Table 1 gives the implied limits of reliability of a result reported to different significant figures.

When zeros appear in a number, they may present a problem when one is trying to determine the number of significant figures. Zeros to the right of the decimal point are always significant if they follow the digits and are not significant if they precede a digit and if the total number is less than one. Thus, 0.072 contains two significant figures; 0.720 contains three significant figures; and 1.072 contains four significant figures. A report of 220 does not indicate whether the measurement was to the nearest tens or to the nearest ones, as the zero is not significant. If there are digits on both sides of the zero, as 202, it is a significant figure. If the zero is followed by a decimal point and digits or zeros, as 220.1, the zero is a significant figure.

Rules for figure retention

1. Retain as many significant figures in data and result as will be necessary to give only one uncertain figure.

EXAMPLE: The number, 36.24 ml, was recorded on a buret whose smallest scale divisions were in tenths. Which are the significant figures?

All figures are significant since 36.2 represents actual scale divisions. The 4 represents interpolation between two scale divisions and is the only one that is uncertain. Another analyst may have read the same setting as 36.23 or 36.25.

2. For a number to have all its digits significant, every digit, except the last, must be correct and the error in the last digit must not be greater than one-half the lowest unit that occupies that space.

EXAMPLE: The number, 36.24, has four significant figures as stated previously. What is the error in this figure?

The 3, 6, and 2 are correct, and the 4 states that the number is closer to 36.24 than it is to 36.235 or 36.245. The lowest unit in the space is 0.01 or $1/100$, and the error is less than or equal to 0.005.

3. In adding or subtracting numbers with differing numbers of digits, retain the significate figures in each term and in the final answer only to the point corresponding to the least number of significant figures occurring after the decimal point.

EXAMPLE: Add 0.0212, 29.64, and 1.056931.

In these three numbers, 0.021*2*, 29.6*4*, and 1.05693*1*, the uncertain figures, 2, 4, and 1, are italicized, and the 4 of 29.64 is farthest to the left. Therefore, the addition would be on the following basis:

$$0.0212 = 0.02$$
$$29.64 = 29.64$$
$$1.056931 = \underline{1.06}$$
$$30.72$$

Since 29.64 only goes into the hundredths column and any following figures are unknown, it is useless to extend the digits of the other terms past the hundredths column.

4. In multiplying and dividing numbers with differing numbers of digits, for practical purposes retain as many significant figures as are found in the factor having the least number of significant figures.

EXAMPLE: What are the significant figures in $0.0211 \times 25.63 \times 1.05881$?

0.0211 has three significant figures
25.63 has four significant figures
1.05881 has six significant figures

In this calculation, 0.0211 is the governing factor, and the problem looks like the following:

$$0.0211 \times 25.6 \times 1.06$$

5. If routine systems for multiplication and division are used, reject all superfluous digits at each stage of the operation.

In using logarithm tables for dividing and multiplying numbers, retain as many figures in the mantissa of the logarithm of each factor as are found in the factors themselves under the preceding rule 3.

EXAMPLE: Calculate $0.0211 \times 25.6 \times 1.06$.

$$\log 0.0211 = 8.324 - 10$$
$$\log 25.6 = 1.408$$
$$\log 1.06 = \underline{0.025}$$
$$\text{Sum of logarithms} = 9.757 - 10 = \text{logarithm of product}$$
$$\text{Antilog } 9.757 - 10 = 0.572$$

RULES FOR ROUNDING OFF NUMBERS

Often times, as the result of mathematical computations, test results are acquired that produce insignificant digits. It then becomes necessary to *round off* the number to the chosen number of significant figures before reporting results. This is done so that one does not infer an accuracy of precision greater than the test is capable of delivering. However, each analyst should follow the same procedures for rounding off to permit consistency in reporting results. The following is the universal system:

1. If the digit to be dropped is less than 5, the preceding figure is not altered.
2. If the digit to be dropped is more than 5, the preceding figure is increased by one.
3. If the digit to be dropped is 5, the preceding figure is increased by one if it is an odd number, and the preceding figure is not altered if it is an even number.

EXAMPLE: The following numbers have been rounded off to one decimal place:

$$3.24 = 3.2$$
$$3.16 = 3.2$$
$$3.15 = 3.2$$
$$3.25 = 3.2$$

If this system is followed by each analyst, no bias will be introduced into calculations of large amounts of data in small quality control procedures.

SCIENTIFIC NOTATION

Often times it is necessary to work with numbers that have a string of zeros behind them or that are just too large to handle efficiently. *Scientific notation* has been devised as a kind of shorthand way of writing such numbers. In this system, the powers of 10 are used. For example, one hundred is 10×10 (100) or 10^2, one thousand is $10 \times 10 \times 10$ (1000) or 10^3, and one million is $10 \times 10 \times 10 \times 10 \times 10 \times 10$ (1,000,000) or 10^6.

To present a larger number in a form that can be easily used and understood, express that number as a number between 1 and 10 multiplied by a power of 10.

EXAMPLE:

$$100 = 1 \times 10^2$$
$$1000 = 1 \times 10^3$$
$$1,000,000 = 1 \times 10^6$$

To convert a number to scientific notation, count the number of places required to move the decimal point to the left to obtain a number between 1 and 10; that number will be the correct positive power of 10.

EXAMPLE:

$$100 = 1 \times 10^2$$
②1

$$1000 = 1 \times 10^3$$
③2 1

$$13,600 = 1.36 \times 10^4$$
④ 3 2 1

$$2,618,000,000 = 2.618 \times 10^9$$
⑨8 7 6 5 4 3 2 1

A number of less than 1 will have a negative power of 10. Count the number of zeros and the first whole number to which the decimal point has been moved to the right to obtain a number between 1 and 10. Said another way, count the number of places the decimal must be moved to the right to obtain a number between 1 and 10. This will be the correct negative power of 10.

EXAMPLE:

$$0.001 = 1 \times 10^{-3}$$
1 2③

$$0.0000431 = 4.31 \times 10^{-5}$$
1 2 3 4⑤

$$0.00000000918 = 9.18 \times 10^{-9}$$
1 2 3 4 5 6 7 8⑨

Multiplication in scientific notation

1. Positive power of 10. To multiply numbers expressed as positive powers of 10, first multiply the numbers (between 1 and 10) that appear to the left of the 10 to a power; then *add* the exponents.

EXAMPLE: $15,100 \times 200,000 = X$

Convert the numbers to scientific notation.

$$15,100 = 1.51 \times 10^4$$
④ 3 2 1

$$200,000 = 2.0 \times 10^5$$
⑤4 3 2 1

Multiply the numbers between 1 and 10.

$$\begin{array}{r} 1.51 \\ \times 2.0 \\ \hline 3.020 \end{array}$$

Add the exponents of 10.

$$10^4 \times 10^5 = 10^{4+5} = 10^9$$

Multiply the two parts.

$$3.02 \times 10^9 = 3,020,000,000$$

2. Negative power of ten. To multiply numbers expressed as negative powers of 10, first multiply the numbers (between 1 and 10) that appear to the left to the 10 to a minus power; then, add the negative exponents.

EXAMPLE: $0.000192 \times 0.000000008 =$

$$0.000192 = 1.92 \times 10^{-4}$$
$$1\,2\,3④$$

$$0.000000008 = 8.0 \times 10^{-9}$$
$$1\,2\,3\,4\,5\,6\,7\,8⑨$$

$$(1.92 \times 10^{-4}) \times (8.0 \times 10^{-9}) = (1.92 \times 8.0) \times (10^{-4} \times 10^{-9}) =$$
$$(1.92 \times 8.0) \times (10^{(-4)+(-9)}) = (1.92 \times 8.0) \times 10^{-13} = 15.36 \times 10^{-13}$$

Division in scientific notation

The same general rules are followed when dividing in scientific notation; except, when dividing exponents with the same base, *subtract* the exponent of the divisor from the exponent of the dividend.

RULE: First divide the numbers (between 1 and 10) that appear to the left of the powers of 10; then, subtract the power of 10 in the denominator from that in the numerator.

EXAMPLE: $540,000 \div 2100 =$

$$540,000 = 5.4 \times 10^5$$
$$⑤4\ \ 3\,2\,1$$

$$2100 = 2.1 \times 10^3$$
$$③2\,1$$

$$(5.4 \times 10^5) \div (2.1 \times 10^3) = (5.4 \div 2.1) \times (10^{5-3}) = (5.4 \div 2.1) \times 10^2 = 2.57 \times 10^2$$

EXAMPLE: $0.00913 \div 0.0000014 =$

$$0.00913 = 9.13 \times 10^{-3}$$
$$1\,2③$$

$$0.0000014 = 1.4 \times 10^{-6}$$
$$1\,2\,3\,4\,5⑥$$

$$\frac{9.13 \times 10^{-3}}{1.4 \times 10^{-6}} = \frac{9.13}{1.4} \times (10^{(-3)-(-6)}) = \frac{9.13}{1.4} \times 10^3 = 6.52 \times 10^3$$

RATIO AND PROPORTION

When one is confronted with the problem of comparing two or more quantities, the ratio and proportion procedure is one good method to use in solving the problem. *Ratio* considers the relative sizes of two numbers. It is found by dividing one number by the number with which it is being compared. A ratio may be expressed in several ways. The ratio of 5 to 4 can be expressed in several ways as seen by the following:

1. Indicated quotient using the division sign is $5 \div 4$.
2. Indicated quotient using the ratio sign is $5:4$.
3. Fraction form is $5/4$.
4. Fraction in decimal form is 1.25.

When a ratio is written in fractional form, it may then be treated like any other fraction. Notice in the preceding ratio (5 to 4) that 5 is being compared to 4, and recall that a ratio is found by dividing one number *by* the number with which it is being compared. In other words, a ratio is expressed exactly as the words describing it are written. *This is very important.*

EXAMPLE: A ratio of 4 to 10 would be written 4:10 (the 4 comes first in the statement; therefore, it also comes first in the written ratio).

EXAMPLE: A ratio of 6 to 2 would be written 6:2.

EXAMPLE: A given test tube contains 6 ml saline and 3 ml serum. What is the saline to serum ratio?

The ratio is 6:3. (The word saline comes first in the question; therefore, the amount corresponding to saline must come first in the written ratio.) What is the serum to saline ratio? The ratio of serum to saline is 3:6. (In this case, the word serum comes first; therefore, the quantity corresponding to serum must come first in the written ratio.)

In reality, a ratio is a quantity of something compared to a quantity of something else. Be careful to ascertain exactly *what* is being compared and then express it in the proper manner.

EXAMPLE: Consider 9 ml saline and 1 ml serum in a test tube (9 ml + 1 ml = 10 ml total volume); the following expressions would be correct:

1. Serum to saline ratio is 1:9 or 1/9.
2. Saline to serum ratio is 9:1 or 9/1.
3. Saline to total volume ratio is 9:10 or 9/10.
4. Total volume to serum ratio is 10:1 or 10/1.

Why each of the written ratios in the preceding example is expressed as it is and what each one means should be understood before continuing.

Proportion is a statement that two ratios are equal. Consider the ratio 1:2. If one ratio is expressed as a fraction, it can be compared to another equal ratio.

$$\frac{1}{2} = \frac{5}{10}$$

The two fractions, 1/2 and 5/10, are the same thing; they are two ratios meaning the same thing, only they are expressed in different ways. But in reality the relationship between the two numbers of each ratio is the same (2 is twice as great as 1, 10 is twice as great as 5).

If one desires to make more (or less) of the same thing *without changing concentration* (or any other kind of relative relationship), it can usually be done using ratio and proportion.

To do the ratio-proportion procedure, use the following format:

$$A \text{ is to } B \text{ as } C \text{ is to } D$$
$$\frac{A}{B} = \frac{C}{D}$$

This format is in the form of an equation. If three of the four values are known, the fourth can be found by calculation.

In setting up the ratio and proportion, the two ratios being compared must be written in the same order and must be in the same units.

EXAMPLE: Using ratio and proportion, if there are 20 gm in 100 ml, how many grams would there be in 20 ml?

Putting the information about one solution in one ratio and the information about the other solution in another ratio would produce the following statement: If there are 20 gm in 100 ml, there would be X gm in 20 ml.

$$\frac{20 \text{ gm}}{100 \text{ ml}} = \frac{X \text{ gm}}{20 \text{ ml}}$$

Solve the equation.

$$100X = 20 \times 20$$
$$100X = 400$$

$$X = \frac{400}{100}$$

$$X = 4 \text{ gm in } 20 \text{ ml}$$

When ratio-proportion problems are written or verbally stated, the order of the values may or may not be in the order for calculation. In setting up the format of the problem, always place the values in each ratio in the same relationship. This is necessary if correct results are expected.

EXAMPLE: If 6 gm of a substance will make 10 ml of a given solution, how many milliliters can be made from 16 gm?

Note that the two ratios are stated differently in this problem. Grams is stated first in the first ratio and milliliters is stated first in the second ratio; however, the problem should be set up as follows:

$$\frac{6 \text{ gm}}{10 \text{ ml}} = \frac{16 \text{ gm}}{X \text{ ml}}$$

Place the value in one ratio directly across the equal sign from the equivalent value in the other ratio, that is, grams across from grams and milliliters across from milliliters, and complete the calculation.

$$\frac{6}{10} = \frac{16}{X}$$

$$6X = 10 \times 16$$
$$6X = 160$$

$$X = \frac{160}{6}$$

$$X = 26.67$$

The 16 gm of substance will make 26.67 ml of solution.

EXAMPLE: How many grams would it take to make 100 ml of solution if 5 gm made 20 ml?

$$\frac{X \text{ gm}}{100 \text{ ml}} = \frac{5 \text{ gm}}{20 \text{ ml}}$$

$$20X = 5 \times 100$$

$$X = \frac{500}{20}$$

$$X = 25$$

Twenty-five grams will make 100 ml of solution.

Practice problems

Add the following:

1. $+81$ and $+16$
2. $+17$ and -21
3. -4 and -22
4. $+6$ and $+7$
5. $+6$ and -7
6. -6 and $+7$
7. -6 and -7

Subtract the following:

8. +7 from +10
9. +4 from −7
10. −14 from +2
11. −6 from +11
12. +36 from +15

13. +3 from +10
14. +6 from −10
15. −3 from +10
16. −3 from −10

Multiply the following:

17. +6 × +8
18. +7 × −2
19. −4 × +10
20. −13 × −3

21. +4 × +5
22. +4 × −5
23. −4 × +5
24. −4 × −5

Divide the following:

25. +66 ÷ +3
26. +6 ÷ −12
27. −15 ÷ +3
28. −20 ÷ −40

29. +20 ÷ +4
30. −20 ÷ +4
31. +20 ÷ −4
32. −20 ÷ −4

State the reciprocal for the following:

33. 10

34. $\dfrac{1}{8}$

35. 1.16

Perform the following computations:

36. +3 − 20 − 7 + 6 − 3 − 2
37. 7 × 6 + 3 ÷ 2 + 17 × 6 − 10 × 3
38. 4 ÷ (3 − 1) + 7 × (6 ÷ 8) − 13
39. [13 × (6 − 1) − 7] + (7 × 2) × {6 + (7 × 3) − [6 + (4 − 8)] − 2}

Multiply the following:

40. $\dfrac{1}{2} \times \dfrac{1}{8}$

41. $\dfrac{3}{6} \times \dfrac{7}{2}$

42. $\dfrac{1}{3} \times 2\dfrac{1}{8}$

Divide the following:

43. $\dfrac{1}{9} \div 3$

44. $\dfrac{2}{6} \div \dfrac{1}{3}$

45. $1\dfrac{3}{8} \div 2\dfrac{1}{2}$

Add the following:

46. $\dfrac{1}{3} + \dfrac{6}{3} + \dfrac{2}{3}$

47. $\dfrac{2}{6} + \dfrac{6}{3} + \dfrac{4}{8}$

48. $1\dfrac{1}{5} + 2\dfrac{3}{15} + 1\dfrac{2}{10}$

Subtract the following:

49. $\dfrac{4}{9} - \dfrac{2}{9}$

50. $\dfrac{6}{5} - \dfrac{6}{10}$

51. $1\dfrac{1}{3} - 5\dfrac{2}{5}$

Give the whole number or fraction that corresponds to the following:

52. 10^7
53. 10^2
54. 10^{-4}
55. 6^5
56. 2^{-3}

57. 10^4
58. 10^{-6}

Perform the following computations:

59. $10^4 + 10^6$

60. $a^2 \times a^6$

61. $b^3 \times c^2$

62. $3^6 - 4^2$

63. $a^9 \div a^6$

64. $\dfrac{a^7}{a^2}$

65. $10^2 + 10^3$

66. $10^{-6} + 10^{-2}$

67. $6^6 \times 6^3$

68. $5^4 \times 5^{-2}$

69. $10^7 \div 10^3$

70. $10^{-4} \div 10^2$

71. $7^6 \times 3^4$

72. Write the ratio 10 to 8 four different ways.

73. In a test tube containing 2 ml serum + 8 ml saline, give the following:
    a. The serum to saline ratio
    b. The saline to serum ratio
    c. The serum to total volume ratio
    d. The total volume to serum ratio
    e. The saline to total volume ratio
    f. The total volume to saline ratio

Complete the following proportions:

74. $\dfrac{1}{2} = \dfrac{X}{8}$

75. $\dfrac{X}{10} = \dfrac{1}{4}$

76. $\dfrac{2}{X} = \dfrac{3}{6}$

77. $\dfrac{4}{20} = \dfrac{5}{X}$

78. If there are 20 gm of substance in 50 ml of solution, how many grams would be present in 10 ml of solution?

79. Given 10 gm of substance and the fact that it takes 2 gm to make 10 ml of solution, how many milliliters solution will the 10 gm make?

80. If there are 30 gm in 100 ml, how many grams would be in 20 ml?

81. Express the following in scientific notation:
    a. 5,000,000
    b. 142,000
    c. 59,000
    d. 0.0000172
    e. 0.00111
    f. 0.00000000291

82. Solve the following using scientific notation:
    a. $913,000 \times 1,260,000$
    b. $26,000 \times 152,000$
    c. 0.000492×0.00127
    d. $520,000 \div 24,000$
    e. $\dfrac{0.0000006}{0.000131}$

Logarithms

A logarithm is the exponent of some number. This number is called the *base*. The abbreviation *log* is generally written instead of *the logarithm of*. The abbreviation log is neither capitalized nor followed by a period and should be used with care.

In working with logarithmic calculations it is important to show properly which numbers are logarithms and which are numbers *corresponding to logarithms*. Since log is the abbreviation for the logarithm of, it is to be written *only* before the number whose logarithm either is known or is to be found. It is *never* written before the logarithm itself. This point should be thoroughly understood. For example, the logarithm of 25 is 1.3979; therefore, write log 25 = 1.3979, because 1.3979 is the logarithm of 25. It would be incorrect to write 25 = log 1.3979, because 25 is not the logarithm of 1.3979.

There are two main systems of logarithms, base 10 and base e. The number 10 is used as the base for one system, and all logarithms of this system are exponents of the number 10. Logarithms to the base 10 are called *common* or *Briggs* logarithms.

In certain special computations, a system of logarithms is used in which the base is the number $2.718281828+$. This number is generally denoted by e. Logarithms to the base e are known as *hyperbolic, Naperian,* or *natural logarithms*. Logarithms in this system are generally designated by the subscript e after the abbreviation log. When no base is designated, common logarithms are usually meant. For example, $\log_e 5$ means the hyperbolic logarithm of 5, and log 5 means the common logarithm of 5.

There are tables for each system of logarithms. However, one type may be found from the other by the use of conversion factors.

EXAMPLE: $20 = 10^{1.30103} = e^{2.99575}$

$$\log 20 = 1.30103$$
$$\log_e 20 = 2.99575$$

$$\frac{\log_e 20}{\log 20} = \frac{2.99575}{1.30103} = 2.303$$

$$\frac{\log 20}{\log_e 20} = \frac{1.30103}{2.99575} = 0.4343$$

These *ratios* always hold true; therefore, to convert common logarithms to natural logarithms, multiply the common logarithm by 2.303. To convert natural logarithms to common logarithms, multiply the natural logarithm by 0.4343.

Here, we will consider the use of common logarithms since these are the ones generally used in laboratory work. It was stated earlier that a logarithm is the exponent of a number called a base. Therefore, the logarithm of a number is the power to which the base must be raised to give that number. Examine the following:

$$1 = 10^{0.0000} \qquad \log 1 = 0.0000$$
$$2 = 10^{0.3010} \qquad \log 2 = 0.3010$$
$$5 = 10^{0.6990} \qquad \log 5 = 0.6990$$
$$9 = 10^{0.9542} \qquad \log 9 = 0.9542$$

$$10 = 10^{1.0000}$$
$$100 = 10^{2.0000}$$
$$1000 = 10^{3.0000}$$
$$0.1 = 10^{-1}$$
$$0.01 = 10^{-2}$$

$$\log 10 = 1.0000$$
$$\log 100 = 2.0000$$
$$\log 1000 = 3.0000$$
$$\log 0.1 = \bar{1}.0000$$
$$\log 0.01 = \bar{2}.0000$$

The logarithm of any number between 1 and 10 is zero plus a decimal, because the logarithm is greater than zero but less than 1. Similarly, the logarithm of any number between 10 and 100 is 1 plus a decimal, because the logarithm is greater than 1 but less than 2. The logarithm of any number between 100 and 1000 is 2 plus a decimal. Likewise, since log 1 is 0 and log 0.1 is −1, the logarithm of any decimal number between 0.1 and 1 is −1 plus a decimal. The log of 0.01 is −2; therefore, the logarithm of any number between 0.01 and 0.1 is −2 plus a decimal. Following this logic, it can be stated that, in general, the logarithm of a number consists of two parts: (1) a whole number, called the *characteristic,* and (2) a decimal fraction, called the *mantissa.* The characteristic of the logarithm may be either positive or negative, depending on whether the number it represents is greater or less than one. However, *the mantissa is always positive!*

DETERMINING THE CHARACTERISTIC
Numbers greater than 1

The characteristic for any number, 1 or greater, is *always zero or a positive number.* The value for the characteristic depends on the location of the decimal point in the original number, and is always one less than the number of digits to the left of the decimal point.

EXAMPLE: Note the characteristic for the following:

$$257 = 2$$
$$2.57 = 0$$
$$25.7 = 1$$
$$2570 = 3$$

Note that the characteristic is obtained by visual inspection of the original number, does not come from a table, and depends solely on the location of the decimal point in the original number.

Numbers less than 1

The characteristic of the logarithm of any number less than 1 is *negative* and is numerically 1 more than the number of zeros *immediately* following the decimal point in the original number. In other words, the negative characteristic is equal to 1 plus the number of decimal places to the first nonzero digit in the fraction. The fact that the characteristic is negative whereas the mantissa is positive may be indicated by the following two means:

1. Writing a minus sign *over* the characteristic will indicate that the characteristic is negative and the mantissa is positive.

EXAMPLE: $\bar{1}.3010$ is the logarithm of 0.2.

This means that the characteristic is −1 and the mantissa is +.3010. It would be incorrect to place a minus sign in front of the characteristic (−1.3010), because this would indicate that both the characteristic and the mantissa are negative; this cannot be correct because the mantissa is *always* positive. Note the characteristics for the following:

$$0.1206 = -1$$

$$0.0001206 = -4$$
$$0.01206 = -2$$
$$0.000001206 = -6$$

while,

$$\log 0.1206 = \overline{1}.0813$$
$$\log 0.0001206 = \overline{4}.0813$$
$$\log 0.01206 = \overline{2}.0813$$
$$\log 0.000001206 = \overline{6}.0813$$

2. A logarithm with a negative characteristic may be changed to a positive form by adding 10 to the characteristic and adding minus 10 after the mantissa. This allows some calculations to be more easily completed.

EXAMPLE: Change the characteristic of $\overline{1}.3010$ to a positive form.

Add 10 to the characteristic.

$$10 + (-1) = 9; 9.3010$$

Then, add -10 after the mantissa.

$$9.3010 - 10$$
$$\overline{1}.3010 = 9.3010 - 10$$

Since 10 is both added and subtracted, the value for the logarithm is not affected. In the logarithm, $9.3010 - 10$, the characteristic has two parts: (1) the positive part, 9, which precedes the mantissa, and (2) the negative part, -10, which follows the mantissa.

The positive part of the characteristic of the logarithm of a decimal number may also be obtained by subtracting the number of zeros between the decimal point and the first significant figure from 9. This number is the positive part of the characteristic. Place -10 after the mantissa. This is the negative part of the characteristic.

EXAMPLE: Find the characteristic for 0.00306.

There are two zeros between the decimal point and the first significant figure, 3. Subtract 2 from 9 and make this the positive part of the characteristic: 7. _____. Add -10: 7. _____ -10. Note the characteristic of the following:

$$\log 0.000432 = \overline{4} \text{ or } 6. \underline{\quad} -10$$
$$\log 0.4320 = \overline{1} \text{ or } 9. \underline{\quad} -10$$
$$\log 0.00432 = \overline{3} \text{ or } 7. \underline{\quad} -10$$

In summary, for numbers less than 1, the characteristic may be expressed two ways:
1. Add 1 to the number of zeros between the decimal point and the first significant figure. This will be a negative number.
2. To change this characteristic to a positive form, add 10 and -10 to the logarithm or subtract the number of zeros between the decimal point and the first significant figure in the number from 9 and add -10 after the mantissa.

Notice again, that the characteristic is found by visual inspection of the number. It does not come from a table and depends entirely on the position of the decimal point in the original number.

DETERMINING THE MANTISSA

As discussed earlier, the mantissa is the decimal part of the logarithm and is always positive. The mantissa cannot be found by visual inspection of the original number. It must be found from a logarithm table and has nothing whatever to do with the position of the decimal in the original number. Although tables given in various texts are called tables of logarithms, they are actually tables of mantissas. The mantissa must be found from the table and then added to the characteristic to form the complete logarithm. Notice that the mantissa given in such tables are usually not preceded by decimal points, because in determining mantissas by means of a table, it is convenient to treat them as whole numbers. However, it should be remembered that a mantissa is entirely decimal and that when used in a logarithm the mantissa should be preceded by a decimal point and a characteristic.

Appendix E is a table of four place logarithms. Tables of logarithms of more than four places exist. These can be used to increase the precision of calculations if desired. The mantissa of any number from 1 to 9999 can be found by using this table. Numbers with more than four significant figures are rounded off to four figures. In determining the number to be used in obtaining a mantissa, do not consider zeros at the beginning or end of any number, with one exception.

This exception being that to find a mantissa in the table, the number for which a mantissa is desired must contain at least three digits, the last two of which may be zero. For numbers with less than three digits simply add enough zeros to the end to produce a three digit number. Remember that the position of the decimal point is determined by the characteristic portion of the logarithm. Hence, the number used for obtaining a mantissa is always three or four digits long, begins with a figure other than zero, and does not contain a decimal point.

Examine the table of four place logarithms in Appendix E. This table consists of a series of vertical columns and horizontal rows. The first two digits of the number for which a logarithm is desired are found in the first column directly under "N." The third digit of the number is found in the row directly to the right of N, and the last digit is found in that portion of the table entitled "proportional parts."

To determine the mantissa of a number, find the first two digits of the number in the left column (N column) of the table. Move across this row to the column headed by the third digit of the number. In logarithms for numbers with less than four digits, record this value as the mantissa of the logarithm. If the number has four digits, record the value found in the column and row of the first three digits of the number and continue to move to the right in the same row to the column of the proportional parts headed by the fourth digit of the number. Add the value found here to the value for the first three figures of the number. This sum is the mantissa of the four-digit number.

EXAMPLE: Consider the following numbers: 5, 50, 0.005, 500.0, and 0.5.

If the decimal point and all preceding and ending zeros are ignored, the number remaining is 5. Add two zeros to make this a three-digit number, that is, 500. Note that the values in the N column range from 10 to 99. Hence, move down this column to 50. Now move across this row to the column headed by 0. Note the value 6990 at this point in the table. This is the mantissa of log 5, log 50, log 0.005, and so on. Each number containing 500 as the significant digits will have a characteristic, which is determined by the position of the decimal point, and a mantissa of .6990.

$$\log 5 = 0.6990$$
$$\log 50 = 1.6990$$
$$\log 0.005 = \bar{3}.6990$$
$$\log 500 = 2.6990$$
$$\log 0.5 = \bar{1}.6990$$

EXAMPLE: Consider the following numbers: 201, 2.01, 0.00201, and 2010.

If the decimal point and the beginning and ending zeros are ignored, the figure 201 is present.

The first two digits of the number (20) are found in the N column, and the digit (1) is found in the top row. Move down the column headed by 1 to the row directly to the right of 20. Find the number .3032. Hence, the mantissa for 201 is .3032.

$$\log 201 = 2.3032$$
$$\log 2.01 = 0.3032$$
$$\log 0.00201 = \bar{3}.3032$$
$$\log 2010 = 3.3032$$

EXAMPLE: Consider the following numbers: 37,950, 37.95, 0.3795, and 0.003795.

Following the instructions for obtaining a mantissa, one should realize that the number to use with each of the above values is 3795. Move down the N column to 37. Move across this row to the column headed by 9. The value at this point in the table is 5786. Continuing in the same row, move to the proportional parts column headed by 5 and find the value 6. Add this to the value for the first three digits of the number.

$$5786 + 6 = 5792$$

Hence, the mantissa for 3795 is .5792. Combine this with the proper characteristic for each number.

$$\log 37,950 = 4.5792$$
$$\log 37.95 = \underline{1}.5792$$
$$\log 0.3795 = \bar{1}.5792 \text{ or } 9.5792 - 10$$
$$\log 0.003795 = \bar{3}.5792 \text{ or } 7.5792 - 10$$

DETERMINATION OF ANTILOGARITHMS

An antilogarithm is the number corresponding to a given logarithm. It is the number for which a logarithm is found.

EXAMPLE: Log 2 = 0.3010; the logarithm of 2 = 0.3010.

The number that gives this logarithm (0.3010) is 2; therefore, 2 is the antilogarithm of 0.3010. The term *antilogarithm of* can be abbreviated to *antilog*.

$$\text{antilog } 0.3010 = 2$$

The antilogarithm may be determined from the logarithm in two ways. One method is to use the logarithm table in reverse order. The second method is to use an antilogarithm table. In both cases the logarithm is divided into the characteristic and the mantissa.

To determine the antilogarithm of the logarithm 0.3010, using the logarithm table, find the mantissa .3010 in the mantissa columns. The two figures from column N that correspond to it are 20; the column heading at the top of the page in the same column with the mantissa is 0. Therefore, our number which corresponds to the mantissa, 3010, is 200.

In the event that the exact mantissa value is not in the table, find the closest mantissa in the columns, that is, find the closest tabular mantissa value, without exceeding the value of the mantissa being worked with. Now move directly to the right and find the value of proportional parts in the same row that, when added to the tabular value, most closely corresponds to the value whose antilogarithm is being sought. Read the first two digits of the antilogarithm from the left most column (N), the third digit from the top row and the fourth digit from the head of the column containing the proportional part used.

EXAMPLE: Find the antilog of 1.8457.

Locate the value in the body of the mantissa table that is closest to, but does not exceed, the mantissa .8457. Move to the left side of this row to the N column and find the number 70, which is the first two digits of the antilogarithm. Note the number at the head of the column containing

.8457. This is the third digit of the antilogarithm. The number at the head of this column is 1. Hence the digits of the antilogarithm of 1.8457 are 701. The characteristic of the logarithm is 1. This indicates that the decimal should be placed two digits from the left, 70.1. Hence the antilog of 1.8457 is 70.1.

EXAMPLE: Find the antilog of 2.7439.

Locate the value in the mantissa table that is closest to, but does not exceed, the mantissa .7439. The closest value in the table is .7435. This figure is found in the 55 row (N) and column headed by 4. Hence, the first three digits of the antilogarithm are 554. Move to the right in this same row in which .7435 is found to the proportional parts section of the table. Find the number that when added to .7435 will give .7439. This number will be 4. The number 4 is found in the column headed by 5. Hence 5 is the fourth digit of the antilogarithm, that is, 5545.

The characteristic of the logarithm is 2. This indicates the position of the decimal point in the digits. Hence the antilog of 2.7439 is 554.5.

To find the antilogarithm using a table of antilogarithms (Appendix F) move down the left most column of the table to the first two digits of the mantissa in question. Move across this row until the column headed by the third digit of the mantissa is reached and record this value. Continue to the right in the same row to the column in the proportional parts portion of the table headed by the fourth digit of the mantissa. Add the value of the proportional part to the antilogarithm of the first three digits. This sum is the basic four place antilogarithm of the logarithm.

EXAMPLE: Find the antilogarithm of the logarithm 0.3010 using the antilogarithm table in Appendix F.

Move down the left column to .30. Move to the right in this row to the column headed by 1. Record 2000. This is the antilogarithm (minus the decimal point) of the mantissa .3010.

The characteristic defines the decimal point. The characteristic is zero. Recall that a positive characteristic is found by subtracting 1 from the number of digits to the left of the decimal point. Therefore, a characteristic of 0 would mean that there was one digit to the left of the decimal point. Therefore, put down the number 2000 and put in the decimal point so that there is one digit to the left of it; the figure would be 2.000.

A negative characteristic is one more than the number of zeros between the decimal point and the first significant figure of the decimal number.

EXAMPLE: Using two methods, find the antilog of the following:

Logarithm	Mantissa	Value from tables	Characteristic	Antilog
3.5453	.5453	3510	3	3510
$\bar{2}$.4116	.4116	2580	$\bar{2}$	0.0258

USE OF LOGARITHMS

Since logarithms are exponents, the rules of exponents are the rules of logarithms.

$$a^b \times a^c = a^{b+c}$$

$$\frac{a^b}{a^c} = a^{b-c}$$

Multiplication using logarithms

To multiply two or more numbers by using logarithms, add the logarithms of the given numbers; then, find the antilog for the resulting sum.

$$3 \times 3$$
$$\log (3 \times 3)$$

$$\log 3 = 0.4771$$
$$\log 3 = \underline{0.4771}$$

Sum of logarithms $= 0.9542 =$ logarithm of product

$$\text{antilog } 0.9542 = 9.0$$
$$3 \times 3 = 9.0$$

If numbers to be multiplied are wholly decimal, the logarithm will contain negative characteristics. These should be converted to the positive form by the addition and subtraction of 10 as described on p. 19. The sum of the -10s must be included as part of the sum of the logarithm. Whenever the negative part of the sum is smaller than the positive part, the indicated subtraction is actually performed to have the logarithm in its simplest form.

EXAMPLE: Find the product of 5.13, 0.0167, 0.91, and 0.00416.

$$\log 52.17 = 1.7174$$
$$\log 0.0143 = 8.1553 - 10$$
$$\log 15 = 1.1761$$
$$\log 0.52 = \underline{9.7160 - 10}$$

Sum of logarithms $= 20.7648 - 20 =$ logarithm of product

$$\begin{array}{r} 20.7648 \\ -20 \\ \hline 0.7648 \end{array}$$

$$\text{antilog } 0.7648 = 5.818$$

If, however, the negative part of the logarithm is the larger and is more than 10, it is reduced to 10 by subtracting the necessary number from it and from the positive part of the logarithm.

EXAMPLE: Find the product of 5.13, 0.0167, 0.91, and 0.00416.

$$\log 5.13 = 0.7101$$
$$\log 0.0167 = 8.2227 - 10$$
$$\log 0.91 = 9.9590 - 10$$
$$\log 0.00416 = \underline{7.6191 - 10}$$

Sum of logarithms $= 26.5109 - 30 =$ logarithm of product

$$\begin{array}{rr} 26.5109 & - 30 \\ -20 & - 20 \\ \hline 6.5109 & - 10 = \bar{4}.5109 = \text{logarithm of product} \end{array}$$

$$\text{antilog } \bar{4}.5109 = 0.0003243$$

Division using logarithms

To divide one number by another using logarithms, first subtract the logarithm of the divisor from the logarithm of the dividend; then, find the antilogarithm for the calculated value.

The logarithm of the dividend should be written first, and below it should be written the logarithm of the divisor. In simple cases the logarithm of the divisor can be subtracted from the logarithm of the dividend without changing the form of either.

$$12 \div 3$$
$$\log (12 \div 3)$$

$$\log 12 = 1.0792$$
$$\log 3 = \underline{0.4771}$$

Difference of logarithms $= 0.6021 =$ logarithm of quotient

$$\text{antilog } 0.6021 = 4.0$$
$$12 \div 3 = 4.0$$

Sometimes it is necessary to change the form of the logarithm of the dividend to obtain the log quotient in a suitable form. The reason for this will become obvious in studying the first setup of the following problem.

EXAMPLE: Divide 4.72 by 16.6.

$$\log 4.72 = 0.6739$$
$$\log 16.6 = 1.2201$$

Before subtracting 1.2201 from 0.6739, it is necessary to add 10 to the 0.6739 and to write −10 after the mantissa to obtain the log quotient in a positive form.

$$\log 4.72 = 10.6739 - 10$$
$$\log 16.6 = \underline{1.2202}$$
$$\text{Difference of logarithms} = 9.4538 - 10 = \text{logarithm of quotient}$$

$$9.4538 - 10 = \overline{1}.4538$$
$$\text{antilog } \overline{1}.4538 = 0.2843$$

Practice problems

Give the logarithm (two ways when applicable) of the following:

1. 5260
2. 5.260
3. 0.00526
4. 0.526
5. 52.60

6. 138.01
7. 0.09927
8. 21.703
9. 5.076
10. 0.00007938

Find the antilogarithm of the following:

11. 6.3222
12. 9.4713 − 10
13. $\overline{2}$.1847
14. 3.6493
15. 6.0294 − 10

16. 1.9513
17. 0.8713
18. $\overline{3}$.7193
19. 3.7193
20. 0.7197

Work the following using logarithms:

21. 76.2 × 0.131 × 0.0021
22. 1010 × 172 × 0.00063
23. 47 ÷ 0.26

24. 176,000 ÷ 5.43

25. $\dfrac{1.76 \times 90{,}000 \times 0.0016}{624 \div 0.000142}$

CHAPTER 3

Conversion factors

Conversion factors are usually single numbers that can be used to do many things. The following are three common uses:

1. To express a quantity of one substance as an equivalent quantity of another substance
2. To allow for differences in color equivalents and molecular weights
3. To combine many calculations into a single process

Often the student uses a factor blindly, following the given instructions, and never bothering to find out why the factor is what it is or from where it came. Having the curiosity to ask and to try to determine why things are as they are is one of the characteristics that separates the good students from the mediocre. The source of factors is no secret, and it should not remain unknown to those who use them.

FACTOR USED TO EXPRESS A QUANTITY OF ONE SUBSTANCE AS AN EQUIVALENT QUANTITY OF ANOTHER SUBSTANCE

The following are some general rules in this use of factors:

1. To calculate a factor of this type, there must be some known basis of comparison between the two substances, for example, their molecular weights.
2. In using a conversion factor in this manner, multiply the known quantity by the conversion factor. The product is the equivalent value.
3. When this type of factor is used, quantities of the two substances must be expressed in the same units, that is, milligram urea nitrogen to milligram urea or gram urea nitrogen to gram urea.

This kind of factor can be obtained at least three ways: (1) look it up in some reference source, (2) use ratio and proportion and set the known relationship against X to 1, and (3) set up the known relationship as a common fraction and convert to a decimal number.

The use of a reference source is excusable if the reference can be easily obtained and if the worker has no professional curiosity.

The use of ratio and proportion may be explained using a very common factor of this type, 2.14 for converting an amount of urea nitrogen to an equivalent amount of urea. The structure of urea is as follows:

$$
\begin{array}{ccc}
\text{H} & \text{O} & \text{H} \\
\diagdown & \| & \diagup \\
\text{N}-\text{C}-\text{N} \\
\diagup & & \diagdown \\
\text{H} & & \text{H}
\end{array}
$$

The molecular weight of urea is calculated by the following procedure:

Element	Number of atoms	Atomic weight	
Carbon	1	12	12
Oxygen	1	16	16
Nitrogen	2	14	28
Hydrogen	4	1	4
		Molecular weight of urea =	60

The molecular weight of the nitrogen in the urea molecule is 28 (2 ×14). Therefore, there are 28 parts of urea nitrogen in 60 parts of urea. The ratio-proportion formula for the determination of the amount of urea equivalent to one part of urea nitrogen is as follows:

$$\frac{60 \text{ parts urea}}{28 \text{ parts urea nitrogen}} = \frac{X \text{ parts urea}}{1 \text{ part urea nitrogen}}$$

$$60 \times 1 = 28X$$
$$28X = 60$$
$$X = 2.14$$

One part of urea nitrogen would be contained in 2.14 parts of urea. Therefore, if the amount of urea nitrogen is multiplied by 2.14, the result equals the amount of urea to which the known quantity of urea nitrogen is equivalent, for example:

Milligrams of urea nitrogen × 2.14 = Milligrams of urea
Grams of urea nitrogen × 2.14 = Grams of urea

This is a use of ratio and proportion in which the known part of a relationship is set against 1 and the desired part of the relationship is set against X. The result of such calculations is the amount of the desired substance that is equal to one unit of the known substance.

$$\frac{60}{28} = \frac{X}{1}$$

Hence, in the preceding example, the answer is the conversion factor used to convert a value for urea nitrogen to an equivalent value for urea.

The important thing is to make what is to be changed equivalent to 1 and to make the desired value equivalent to X. Note that if the entire ratio-proportion setup is turned over, the answer will remain the same.

$$\frac{60}{28} = \frac{X}{1} \qquad\qquad\qquad \frac{28}{60} = \frac{1}{X}$$
$$X = 2.14 \qquad\qquad\qquad\qquad X = 2.14$$

The third method to obtain a factor is to write the known relationship as a common fraction and convert this to a decimal number. To arrive at a conversion factor in this manner, divide the number that represents the comparative amount of the existing material into the number that represents the comparative amount of the desired material. This answer is the conversion factor. Caution should be observed in using the known relationship properly. This method can be used to produce two conversion factors from one relationship between two substances. Be sure that the conversion factor calculated is the one that will convert the value for the existing material to the value for the desired material and not vice versa. Use common sense.

EXAMPLE: Find the concentration of NaCl that would be equivalent to 100 mg/dl Cl.

The concentration of Cl is the existing value, whereas the concentration of NaCl is the desired value.

1. Study of a reference shows that the atomic weight of chlorine to be 35.5 and the molecular weight of sodium chloride to be 58.5.
2. The number representing NaCl is greater than the number representing Cl.

$$58.5 > 35.5$$

3. Therefore, if one wants to change 100 mg/dl Cl into an equivalent amount of NaCl, the answer must be greater than the concentration of chlorine present.

$$100 \text{ mg/dl Cl} = X \text{ mg/dl NaCl}$$
$$X \text{ must be} > 100 \text{ mg/dl}$$

4. To get a larger number, one must multiply the amount of Cl present by a factor greater than 1.

$$100 \text{ mg/dl Cl} \times \text{factor} = X \text{ mg/dl NaCl}$$
$$\text{factor must be} > 1$$

5. To get a factor greater than 1 divide the larger number of the comparison by the smaller, that is, 58.5 ÷ 35.5.

$$\frac{58.5}{35.5} = 1.65$$

$$1.65 > 1$$

6. The factor used to change a concentration of chlorine to an equivalent concentration of sodium chloride is 1.65.

7. To use the factor, multiply the observed value by the factor to get the equivalent value.

$$100 \text{ mg/dl Cl} \times 1.65 = 165 \text{ mg/dl NaCl}$$
$$165 > 100$$

EXAMPLE: Change 200 mg/dl NaCl to mg/dl Cl.

1. The molecular weight of NaCl is 58.5 and the molecular weight of Cl is 35.5

$$\text{NaCl} = 58.5$$
$$\text{Cl} = 35.5$$

2. The number representing Cl is smaller than the number representing NaCl.

$$35.5 < 58.5$$

3. Therefore, the final amount of Cl must be less than the 200 mg/dl NaCl.

$$200 \text{ mg/dl NaCl} = X \text{ mg/dl Cl}$$
$$X \text{ must be} < 200 \text{ mg/dl}$$

4. To get a smaller amount, multiply the amount of NaCl by a factor of less than 1.

$$200 \text{ mg/dl NaCl} \times \text{factor} = \text{mg/dl Cl}$$
$$\text{factor must be} < 1$$

5. To get a factor of less than 1, divide the smaller comparative number by the larger, that is, 35.5 ÷ 58.5.

$$\frac{35.5}{58.5} = 0.61$$

$$0.61 < 1$$

$$200 \text{ mg/dl NaCl} \times 0.61 = 122 \text{ mg/dl Cl}$$
$$122 < 200$$

This method is actually a short version of the ratio-proportion procedure. The right side of the setup, that is, $X/1$, is used for the factor. Note that when a number is used as a numerator over 1, the resulting fraction is equal to the number itself. An important consideration of this method of calculating factors is that because only part of the ratio-proportion procedure is used, this relationship *cannot* be turned over without changing the factor.

$$\frac{58.5}{35.5} = 1.65$$

turned over

$$\frac{35.5}{58.5} = 0.61$$

IN REVIEW:

1. Conversion factors may be figured by using ratio and proportion.
2. Conversion factors may be figured by using only the known relationship as a fraction and converting this to a decimal number.

If the ratio-proportion procedure is to be used, put down the known relationship, fill in the opposite side of the problem, making the substance to be changed equivalent to 1, and solve for X; the answer is the factor. If this relationship is turned upside down, the same answer will still be received providing the ratio-proportion procedure is correct.

In using the comparative relationships only, always put the number that corresponds to the *basis* for comparison or change (that is, the standard or the substance being changed) on the bottom and the other number on the top; then, reduce the fraction. The resulting answer is the factor. This type of problem *may not* be turned upside down without changing the result.

EXAMPLE: What is the conversion factor for converting milligrams of urea to milligrams of urea nitrogen?

$$\frac{28 \text{ urea nitrogen}}{60 \text{ urea}} = \frac{X \text{ urea nitrogen}}{1 \text{ urea}}$$

$$60X = 28$$
$$X = 0.467$$
$$\text{mg urea} \times 0.467 = \text{mg urea nitrogen}$$

EXAMPLE: What is the conversion factor for converting mg/dl Cl to mg/dl NaCl?

$$\frac{58.5 \text{ NaCl}}{35.5 \text{ Cl}} = \frac{X \text{ NaCl}}{1 \text{ Cl}}$$

$$35.5X = 58.5$$
$$X = 1.65$$
$$\text{mg/dl Cl} \times 1.65 = \text{mg/dl NaCl}$$

EXAMPLE: What is the conversion factor for converting grams of NaCl to grams of Cl?

$$\frac{35.5 \text{ Cl}}{58.5 \text{ NaCl}} = \frac{X \text{ Cl}}{1 \text{ NaCl}}$$

$$58.5X = 35.5$$
$$X = 0.61$$
$$\text{gm NaCl} \times 0.61 = \text{gm Cl}$$

FACTORS USED TO ALLOW FOR DIFFERENCES IN COLOR EQUIVALENTS OR MOLECULAR DIFFERENCES

Frequently, one reaction may be used to test for a variety of compounds, and, if colorimetry is used to evaluate the test results, allowances need to be made in the color equivalent values obtained. The test for sulfonamides is a good example. All the drugs in this group contain the sulfonamide group ($-SO_2NH_2$), which participates in a diazo reaction with the subsequent formation of a colored compound. The sulfa compounds have similar chemical properties but differ from each other in molecular structure and weight. Colorimetry values are often considered to vary directly with the molecular weights of the test materials. In theory, the particular drug being measured should also be used for the standard because some authors state that the intensity of color produced by a given amount of the different drugs is not always in the calculated proportions to their molecular weights. However, such deviations are usually small, and their consideration is generally not worthwhile. In cases in which a substance different from that being measured is used for the standard, the formula for the factor is as follows:

$$\text{Conversion factor} = \frac{\text{Mol wt of drug being measured}}{\text{Mol wt of drug used as standard}}$$

To express a quantity of one substance as an equivalent quantity of another substance, a known relationship is needed between the two substances in question. Again the molecular weights may be used. Using this known relationship, it is possible to work these problems in the same two ways discussed previously in this chapter: (1) by using the ratio-proportion procedure, in which case the ratio proportion is set up with a comparison of one part standard, and (2) by using the two comparative figures and dividing the molecular weight of the standard into the molecular weight of the drug in question.

EXAMPLE: If one were measuring Sulfanilamide and had used Sulfathiazole as the standard, what would be the conversion factor?

$$\text{Mol wt of Sulfanilamide} = 172$$
$$\text{Mol wt of Sulfathiazole} = 255$$

$$\frac{172}{255} = \frac{X}{1}$$

$$255X = 172$$
$$X = 0.674 = \text{Conversion factor}$$

One would then multiply the answer derived in the test by the conversion factor.

RULE: When using only the molecular weights, always put the basis for comparison (or change) on the bottom, which in this case is the standard, the reason for this being the same as before (see pp. 26-28).

FACTORS USED TO COMBINE MANY CALCULATIONS INTO A SINGLE PROCESS

The factors under this heading need little explanation. The factor is simply the reduction of two or more calculations into a single number.

In any situation in which there are several steps in a calculation that are always the same, one may reduce them to a single factor to be used each time, thereby reducing time and work.

One example of this kind of factor is the number 50, used to determine the manual white blood cell count. This procedure is used to ascertain the concentration of white blood cells in a sample of blood. The results are reported as the number of white blood cells per cubic millimeter. To count all the white blood cells in 1 mm³ of blood would be unreasonably difficult for routine work, so a much smaller volume of blood is used. Several factors are used to make the results of the count equivalent to the number of white blood cells per cubic millimeter. The volume of blood is reduced or changed in three ways: (1) the blood is diluted, (2) a greater area than 1 mm² is counted, and (3) a depth of blood much less than 1 mm is used. Since each of these results in a volume other than 1 mm³, there are three different factors: (1) dilution, (2) area, and (3) depth.* With the usual dilution (1:20) and the area counted (4 mm²) on a standard counting

---

*These are explained in detail in Chapter 11.

chamber (depth 0.1 mm) with Neubauer ruling, the total number of cells can be calculated by the following procedure:

$$\text{Cells counted} \times \text{Dilution factor} \times \text{Area factor} \times \text{Depth factor} = \text{Cells/mm}^3$$
$$\text{Cells counted} \times 20 \times \tfrac{1}{4} \times 10 = \text{Cells/mm}^3$$

To do this each time would be time consuming and pointless. Since the three factors are always the same, the three individual factors may be combined into a single number.

$$\text{Cells counted} \times (20 \times \tfrac{1}{4} \times 10) = \text{Cells/mm}^3$$
$$\text{Final factor} = 20 \times \tfrac{1}{4} \times 10 = 50$$
$$\text{Cells counted} \times 50 = \text{Cells/mm}^3$$

If correction factors are constantly changing, it is of no benefit to figure a final factor, however, such a factor may save a great deal of time and effort if the intermediate factors are constant.

EXAMPLE: To convert mg/dl Cl to mEq/l the following formula may be used. What factor could be used instead?

$$\text{mEq/l} = \frac{\text{mg/dl} \times 10}{35.5}$$

The 10 and the 35.5 are constant; therefore, they may be converted to the following factor:

$$\text{mEq/l} = \text{mg/dl} \times \frac{10}{35.5}$$

$$\text{mEq/l} = \text{mg/dl} \times 0.282 \text{ (factor)}$$

CORRECTION FOR VARIATION IN PROCEDURE QUANTITIES

There are several situations in laboratory work in which a different quantity is used from the one described in a procedure. In such cases this difference must be considered in the calculations relating to the reporting of the results. The use of data from another test, collecting insufficient sample, accidental destruction of some part of a sample, and the use of equipment designed for another procedure are all examples of this situation.

The calculations relating to this sort of correction can be summarized by the following general rule: *Divide by what was used and multiply by what should have been used.*

EXAMPLE: A procedure for sodium determination calls for 5 ml urine. However, the amount of specimen sent to the laboratory consisted of only 3.5 ml.

To complete this test, 3 ml of urine were diluted with 2 ml of distilled water to make a total volume of 5 ml. The sodium concentration in this volume was 40 mEq/l. This result must be corrected for the insufficient sample volume. Correct for this by using the rule: Divide by what was used and multiply by what should have been used. Three milliliters of urine were used; divide 40 mEq/l by 3.

$$\frac{40}{3} = 13.33$$

Multiply by what should have been used, that is, 5 ml of urine.

$$13.33 \times 5 = 66.65$$

There are two ways of thinking about the calculations involved in the use of this rule. In one sense, this is a ratio-proportion problem; it could also be viewed as a correction for a dilution.

Set this up as a ratio-proportion problem. If 3 ml of urine has a concentration of 40 mEq/l, how many mEq/l would be in 5 ml of urine?

$$\frac{3}{40} = \frac{5}{X}$$

$$3X = 200$$
$$X = 66.65 \text{ mEq/l}$$

If one considers that a dilution was made of the original sample, correction for this should be made with the test results. A 3/5 dilution was made of the sample. To correct for this, multiply the results by the reciprocal of the dilution, that is, 5/3 (see Chapter 8); by doing this, one is dividing by what was used and multiplying by what should have been used.

$$\frac{5}{3} \times 40 = 66.65 \text{ mEq/l}$$

Practice problems

1. What is the factor for converting Br to NaBr?
2. What is the factor for converting NaCl to Na?
3. Using a factor, convert 300 mg/dl Cl to mg/dl NaCl.
4. Using a factor, convert 500 mg/dl NaBr to mg/dl Br.
5. Sulfadiazine is being measured. The answer, from a curve setup using Sulfamerazine as the standard, was 50 mg/dl. Using a factor, derive the correct answer. Molecular weight of sulfadiazine is 250, and molecular weight of sulfamerazine is 264.
6. In a certain procedure there are four constant correction factors: 20, 1/10, 1/5, and 100. Derive a single factor.
7. A test is being run that calls for 1 ml of spinal fluid. Only 0.4 ml is available for testing. The answer obtained is 120 mg/dl. What answer should be reported?
8. A procedure is being done that calls for 5 ml undiluted urine. Three milliliters of a 1/10 dilution of urine is available for use. The answer is 30 mg/dl. What should be reported?

CHAPTER 4

Systems of measure

METRIC SYSTEM

The United States of America is one of the few countries in the world that does not use the metric system of measure. This system is compatible with mathematics using decimals. Since the decimal-based system of mathematics is usually used in the laboratory, all nonmetric measurements should be converted to the metric system for use in laboratory procedures and calculations.

The metric system has many basic standards of physical phenomena. This chapter will consider three of these standards: the meter, the gram, and the liter. The meter is a basic unit of linear measure. Multiples of this standard are used as a measure of area and volume. The gram is a standard base unit of mass; in other words, the gram is used to measure how much matter is contained in some object. The liter is a conveinent unit of volume that is commonly used in lieu of the decimeter cubed.

These basic units are of little practical improvement over the basic units of other systems. The advantage of the metric system is in the method used to divide or multiply the units. The fractional parts of the basic units are made according to decimal fractions; that is, larger or smaller units are derived by multiplying the basic standard by some power of 10. The multiples of the basic standards are assigned a prefix and a symbol that are constant for all standards. Study of Table 2 should aid in understanding this. Any of the multiples may be used with any basic metric standard. The prefix is added to the standard name. For example, 1 km is equal to 1000 m, 1 ml is equal to 1/1000 l, and 1 μg is equal to 1/1,000,000 gm.

The basic standards are equivalent to the multiple 10^0, or 1, and do not carry a prefix.

Table 3 contains examples of some of the more common units of measure used in the biological laboratory. Notice that the table does not include all possible combinations of the basic standards and prefixes. This is simply because all combinations are unnecessary for the convenient use of the metric system.

The units of measure in Table 3 and the prefixes in Table 2 conform to the latest recommendations of the International Union of Pure and Applied Chemistry and the International Federation for Clinical Chemistry.

There are several other units of measure that are based on the metric system but that do not strictly conform to the rules of the system. Some of these units are designed to meet a specialized need. The most common example of this is the Angström unit. This is a unit of length nearly equal to 0.1 nanometers. This unit of measure was developed for use in the study of wavelengths of light. It is also a convenient unit of measure for use with molecules and cell organelles.

There are other units commonly seen in biological laboratories that do not meet all the current rules of the metric system. These units developed through tradition and specific application of some of the basic concepts during the original development of the metric system. The units, micron, lambda, and gamma, are examples of such development.

Table 2

Multiple name	Power of 10	Decimal	Prefix	Symbol
Trillion	10^{12}	1,000,000,000,000.0	Tera	T
Billion	10^9	1,000,000,000.0	Giga	G
Million	10^6	1,000,000.0	Mega	M
Thousand	10^3	1000.0	Kilo	k
Hundred	10^2	100.0	Hecto	h
Ten	10^1	10.0	Deca	da
Basic unit	10^0	1.0	(No prefix)	
One-tenth	10^{-1}	0.1	Deci	d
One-hundredth	10^{-2}	0.01	Centi	c
One-thousandth	10^{-3}	0.001	Milli	m
One-millionth	10^{-6}	0.000001	Micro	μ
One-billionth	10^{-9}	0.000000001	Nano	n
One-trillionth	10^{-12}	0.000000000001	Pico	p
One-quadrillionth	10^{-15}	0.000000000000001	Femto	f
One-quintillionth	10^{-18}	0.000000000000000001	Atto	a

Table 3

Multiple	Mass	Length	Volume
1000	Kilogram (kg)	Kilometer (km)	Kiloliter (kl)
1 (basic standard)	Gram (gm or g)	Meter (m)	Liter (l)
1/10	Decigram (dg)	Decimeter (dm)	Deciliter (dl)
1/100	Centigram (cg)	Centimeter (cm)	Centiliter (cl)
1/1000	Milligram (mg)	Millimeter (mm)	Milliliter (ml)
1/1,000,000	Microgram (μg)	Micrometer (μm)	Microliter (μl)
1/1,000,000,000	Nanogram (ng)	Nanometer (nm)	Nanoliter (nl)
1/10,000,000,000		Angström (Å)	
1/1,000,000,000,000	Picogram (pg)	Picometer (pm)	Picoliter (pl)

These are the traditional names of micrometer, microliter, and microgram and have the symbols μ, λ, and γ, respectively. The proper name for such units of 1/1,000,000 basic standard includes the prefix micro and the standard name. The symbols for these units are composed of μ and the symbol of the basic standard (see Table 3). The use of the traditional units is technically incorrect but functionally useful. The laboratory worker should recognize both forms of these units and know their values.

Another traditional usage of the metric system that is not considered correct is the use of combinations of prefixes. Units such as millimicrometer refer to the product of the combination of prefixes. Milli refers to 1/1000 and micro to 1/1,000,000; hence, millimicro refers to 1/1000 × 1/1,000,000 or 1/1,000,000,000, so millimicrometer is a unit denoting 1/1,000,000,000 meter. This, of course, is equal to one nanometer. The use of such combinations of prefixes should be recognized, understood, and discouraged. The established prefixes in Table 2 provide ample latitude in the development of acceptable units for almost any situation.

MEASUREMENT CONVERSIONS

Calculations in the biological laboratory frequently involve the conversion of one unit of measure to another. For instance, how many nanograms are in 0.0078 gm, how many milliliters are equal to 7 oz or how many ounces are in $^2/_3$ lb.

One important principle to remember in converting one unit of measure to another is that the two units must be measures of the same property. For instance, all units of length are compatible, or all units of mass are compatible, but a unit of length is not compatible with a unit of mass. One exception to this consideration is the conversion between units of weight and units of mass. Technically, weight is the force with which a body is attracted toward the earth, and mass is the amount of matter contained within a body. Such measures as pounds, ounces, and grains are units of weight. Such measures as grams, kilograms, and milligrams are units of mass. These units are all commonly used in the same manner in the biological laboratory; so within the context of this work, units of mass and weight are compatible.

Probably the easiest method to use to convert measurements from one unit to another is to develop a conversion factor between the two units in question. The calculation of factors within the metric system is particularly simple because of the decimal base of compatible units.

The conversion factor between two compatible units of the metric system can be calculated by manipulation of the exponents of 10 indicated by the prefixes of the units of measure involved. Note the exponent of 10 for each prefix of the metric units in Table 2. Using the rules for subtraction of positive and negative numbers, subtract the exponent of the desired unit from the exponent of the existing unit. Ten to the power of this result is equal to the conversion factor. This number is then converted to a decimal number and used to convert one unit of metric measure to another. To obtain a value in the desired units multiply the value in the existing units by this factor.

EXAMPLE: How many nanograms are equal to 0.0078 mg?

The existing unit prefix is milli (10^{-3}), and the desired unit prefix is nano (10^{-9}).

$$-3 - (-9) = -3 + 9 = 6$$

Hence

$$10^{-3} \div 10^{-9} = 10^6$$

The factor for converting milligrams to nanograms is $10^6 = 1,000,000$; hence, 0.0078 mg $\times$ 1,000,000 = 7800 ng.

EXAMPLE: How many milligrams are equal to 0.0078 ng?

The existing unit prefix is nano (10^{-9}), and the desired unit prefix is milli (10^{-3}).

$$-9 - (-3) = -9 + 3 = -6$$

Hence

$$10^{-9} \div 10^{-3} = 10^{-6}$$

The factor for converting nanograms to milligrams is 10^{-6} or 0.000001; hence, 0.0078 ng $\times$ 0.000001 = 0.0000000078 mg.

EXAMPLE: How many liters equal 38,967 ml?

The existing unit is 10^{-3}, and the desired unit is 10^0.

$$-3 - 0 = -3$$

Hence

$$10^{-3} \div 10^0 = 10^{-3} \div 1 = 10^{-3}$$

The factor for converting milliliters to liters is 10^{-3} or 0.001; hence, 38,967 ml $\times$ 0.001 = 38.967 l.

EXAMPLE: How many kilometers would it take to make 46,520 dm?

The existing unit is 10^{-1}, and the desired unit is 10^3.

$$-1 - (+3) = -4$$

Hence

$$10^{-1} \div 10^3 = 10^{-4}$$

The factor for converting decimeters to kilometers is 10^{-4} or 0.0001; hence, $46,520 \times 0.0001 = 4.652$ km.

Another method of conversion from one unit of measure to another in the metric system involves the use of the decimal multiples indicated by the prefixes of the unit involved. To determine the conversion factor follow the procedure indicated below:

1. Determine the decimal multiple indicated by the prefixes involved.
2. Arrange one number under the other with the decimal points aligned one directly over the other.
3. Mark through all zeros that are *both* between a 1 and the decimal point *and* directly over or under another zero.
4. Under these two figures, write a zero under each column in which there is a zero left unmarked.
5. If the two original numbers do not have the decimal point on the same side, add one more zero (in the place of the decimal point).
6. Place a one to the left of this row of zeros and a decimal point to the right; this is the conversion factor.

EXAMPLE: Find the *factor* for converting milligrams to nanograms.

The decimal multiple for milli is 0.001, and the decimal multiple for nano is 0.000000001. Place decimals over each other and mark out zeros that are *both* between a one and the decimal point *and* directly over or under another zero as follows:

$$0.0\!\!\not0\!\!\not01$$
$$0.0\!\!\not0\!\!\not00000001$$

Under these two figures, write a zero under each column in which there is a zero left unmarked as follows:

$$0.0\!\!\not0\!\!\not01$$
$$0.0\!\!\not0\!\!\not00000001$$
$$\overline{000000}$$

The decimal points of the original numbers are on the same side; therefore, place a 1 to the left of this row of zeros and a decimal point to the right.

$$0.0\!\!\not0\!\!\not01$$
$$0.0\!\!\not0\!\!\not00000001$$
$$\overline{1000000.} = \text{factor} = 1,000,000$$

EXAMPLE: Find the *factor* for converting decaliter to deciliter.

The multiple for deca is 10, and the multiple for deci is 0.1.

$$10.$$
$$\underline{0.1}$$
$$0$$

The decimal points of the original numbers are on different sides; therefore, one more zero is added.

$$10$$
$$\underline{0.1}$$
$$100. = \text{factor} = 100$$

EXAMPLE: Find the *factor* for converting meters to millimeters.

The multiple for meter, the basic unit, is 1.0, and the multiple for milli is 0.001.

$$\frac{1.0}{0.001}$$
$$1000. \quad = \text{factor} = 1000$$

Note that the zero after the 1 in the decimal multiple for the basic unit is not used since it does not fall *between* a 1 and a decimal point. Also, one more zero is added since the decimal points in the original numbers are not on the same side.

EXAMPLE: Find the *factor* for converting decaliters to kiloliters.

The multiple for deca is 10, and the multiple for kilo is 1000.

$$\frac{10.0}{1000.}$$
$$100. \quad = \text{factor} = 100$$

EXAMPLE: Find the *factor* to convert gram to decagram.

The multiple for gram is 1.0, and the multiple for deca is 10.0.

$$\frac{1.0}{10.0}$$
$$10. \quad = \text{factor} = 10$$

EXAMPLE: Find the *factor* to convert centimeters to milliliters.

These are incompatible units of measure and conversion between them cannot validly be made.

Factors developed in the above manner are used in two different ways, depending on the direction of the conversion. It is important to know which way to use the factors in solving a particular problem. When using the factor to convert a larger unit to a smaller unit, multiply the larger unit by the factor. When using the factor to convert a smaller unit to a larger unit, divide the smaller unit by the factor.

EXAMPLE: Convert 0.22 mg to micrograms.

Since 1 mg is larger than 1 μg, *multiply* the existing larger value by the factor. The multiple of milli is 0.001, and the multiple of micro is 0.000001.

$$\frac{0.001}{0.000001}$$
$$1000. \quad = \text{factor} = 1000$$
$$0.22 \text{ mg} \times 1000 = 220 \ \mu\text{g}$$

EXAMPLE: Convert 1053 cl to decaliters.

Since 1 cl is smaller than 1 dal, *divide* the existing smaller value by the factor. The multiple for centi is 0.01, and the multiple for deca is 10.0.

$$\frac{0.01}{10.0}$$
$$1000. \quad = \text{factor} = 1000$$
$$1053 \text{ cl} \div 1000 = 1.053 \text{ dal}$$

REMEMBER: *Larger to smaller, multiply; smaller to larger, divide.* LSM or SLD, *notLSD*.

NONMETRIC SYSTEMS OF MEASURE

Nonmetric systems of measure are much more complex in their organization than the decimal based system of the metric system. There is little consistency in the relative magnitude of the units of measure of any one property. Appendix I gives the relative values of most of the systems and units of measure used in the laboratories in the United States. Tradition, established procedures, and other factors may require that laboratory personnel use nonmetric units of measure. However, the metric system should be used whenever possible because it has much greater compatibility with decimal-based mathematics and is used more in other countries.

The system of measure used in this country is a conglomeration of older systems. This system is usually called the English system, as most of the system was used in England at the time of the development of the United States. However, today, the system of measure used in the United States has several significant differences from the British system of measure that was official in England until the 1970s. These differences are evident in Appendix I.

As a matter of practical consideration, there are a few units that are much used in this country. The following units of measure are the ones most commonly seen in the laboratory. The memorization of these units will save the laboratory worker time and energy in calculations involving measurement. Again the values of many other units of measure are found in Appendix I.

1 gram = 15.4 grains
1 avoirdupois ounce = 28.35 grams
1 avoirdupois pound = 16 avoirdupois ounces
1 kilogram = 2.2 pounds
1 fluidram = 3.7 milliliters
1 fluidounce = 29.6 milliliters
1 gallon = 128.0 fluidounces
1 inch = 2.54 centimeters
1 foot = 0.305 meters

To convert values of the nonmetric system from one unit to another use the ratio-proportion procedure. This is true for conversions between two units of a nonmetric system and between one nonmetric unit and one metric unit of measure.

EXAMPLE: A patient is 6 feet 1 inch tall. How tall is this patient in centimeters? In meters? Using ratio and proportion, set up the problem: 1 foot is to 12 inches as 6 feet are to X inches.

$$\frac{1 \text{ foot}}{12 \text{ inches}} = \frac{6 \text{ feet}}{X \text{ inches}}$$

$$1X = 12 \times 6$$
$$X = 72 \text{ inches}$$

He was 6 feet 1 inch tall; hence, $72 + 1 = 73$ inches. The relationship between inches and centimeters is as follows: 1 inch is to 2.54 cm as 73 inches are to X centimeters.

$$\frac{1 \text{ inch}}{2.54 \text{ cm}} = \frac{73 \text{ inches}}{X \text{ cm}}$$

$$1X = 2.54 \times 73$$
$$X = 185.4 \text{ cm}$$

The multiple of centi is 10^{-2}, and the multiple of meter is 10^0; hence, $-2 - 0 = -2$. The factor to convert centimeters to meters is 10^{-2} or 0.01; hence, $185.4 \text{ cm} \times 0.01 = 1.854 \text{ m}$.

EXAMPLE: How many grams are there in 6 lb?

This problem may be done at least two different ways. From the common units above, a relationship between pounds and kilograms and one between kilogram and grams is shown. Therefore pounds can be converted to kilograms, and then kilograms can be converted to grams using a factor. Also a relationship is shown between pounds and ounces and between ounces and grams;

therefore, pounds can be converted to ounces, and ounces can be converted to grams. Using ratio and proportion, set up the problem.

Method 1

Step 1. 1 kg is to 2.2 lb as X kg are to 6 lb.

$$\frac{1 \text{ kg}}{2.2 \text{ lb}} = \frac{X \text{ kg}}{6 \text{ lb}}$$

$$2.2X = 6$$
$$X = 2.727 \text{ kg}$$
$$6 \text{ lb} = 2.727 \text{ kg}$$

Step 2. Convert kilograms to grams. The multiple of kilo is 1000, and the multiple of gram is 1.0.

$$\frac{1.0}{1000.} \quad \frac{1000.0}{} = \text{factor} = 1000$$

A larger unit is being converted to a smaller unit; therefore, multiply the larger value by the factor.

$$2.727 \text{ kg} \times 1000 = 2727 \text{ gm}$$

$$6 \text{ lb} = 2727 \text{ gm}$$

Method 2

Step 1. 1 lb = 16 oz; therefore, 1 lb is to 16 oz as 6 lb are to X oz.

$$\frac{1 \text{ lb}}{16 \text{ oz}} = \frac{6 \text{ lb}}{X \text{ oz}}$$

$$X = 6 \times 16$$
$$X = 96 \text{ oz}$$

$$6 \text{ lb} = 96 \text{ oz}$$

Step 2. 1 oz = 28.35 gm; therefore, 1 oz is to 28.35 gm as 96 oz is to X gm.

$$\frac{1 \text{ oz}}{28.35 \text{ gm}} = \frac{96 \text{ oz}}{X \text{ gm}}$$

$$1X = 2721.6 \text{ gm}$$

$$6 \text{ lb} = 2721.6 \text{ gm}$$

This problem may also be solved in one step if the relationship between grams and pounds is known.

Practice problems

1. A patient weighs 210 pounds. What is this patient's weight in kilograms?
2. To figure surface area, one needs the patient's height in centimeters. A patient is 5 feet 10 inches tall. What is this patient's height in centimeters? In meters?
3. Express the following:
   a. 600 mg as decigrams
   b. 1500 μg as centigrams
   c. 0.6 dg as nanograms
   d. 5000 cg as kilograms
   e. 0.36 kg as milligrams
4. Express as milliliters:
   a. 1000 lambda (λ)
   b. 50 dl
   c. 6 dal
5. 6 μm equals how many centimeters?

6. 6×10^{-6} gm is equivalent to which of the following:
   a. 0.00006 gm
   b. 0.00006 mg
   c. 0.006 gm
   d. 0.006 mg
7. 200 lb equal how many grams?
8. 16 gm equal how many ounces?
9. 300 oz equal how many gallons?
10. Convert the following:
    a. 600 μl to deciliters
    b. 3 dag to centigrams
    c. 3 yards to meters
    d. 15 oz to pounds
    e. 2.5 gallons to liters

CHAPTER 5

Temperature conversions

Three scales are commonly used in laboratories to measure the potential of a substance to lose heat, that is, temperature. These scales are Fahrenheit, Kelvin, and Celsius. The Celsius scale is frequently and erroneously referred to as the centigrade scale. Fig. 5-1 shows the relative temperatures of four natural phenomena.

The Celsius and Kelvin scales are divided into units, called *degrees,* of equal magnitude. The difference in these scales is in the position of the zero point. In the Kelvin scale the zero point is the theoretical temperature of no further heat loss, that is, absolute zero. The Celsius scale has the freezing point of water as the zero point. Water freezes at $+273°K$; hence, $0°C = 273°K$ or $0°K = -273°C$. The Fahrenheit scale is divided into degrees of a different magnitude from the other two. Also, the zero point of this scale is different from the others.

In the United States, laboratory procedures are written using any one of these three temperature scales. Often it becomes necessary to convert temperature values from one scale to another.

Conversion between the Celsius and Kelvin scales is relatively simple. To convert degrees Kelvin to degrees Celsius, subtract 273 from the value in degrees Kelvin. To convert degrees Celsius to degrees Kelvin, add 273 to the value in degrees Celsius.

$$°K = °C + 273$$
$$°C = °K - 273$$

This simplicity is possible because the units of the two scales are equal. A $100°$ temperature change would be the same with either scale. Water, at standard pressure, boils at $100°C$ or $373°K$. The difference between the boiling point and freezing point of water is $100°$, using either the Kelvin or Celsius scale.

Conversions between the Celsius and Fahrenheit scales are somewhat more complicated. The Fahrenheit scale has the zero point set at the lowest temperature attainable from a mixture of table salt and ice. $100°F$ was set at the body temperature of a small animal. This scale was later standardized against the Celsius scale, the original standards were variable. The freezing point of water is $32°F$, whereas the boiling point of water at standard pressure is $212°F$. This results in degree increments of a different magnitude from the other two scales. Hence, the conversion between the Fahrenheit scale and the other scales is somewhat complicated. Table 4 shows the boiling and freezing point of water in the Fahrenheit and Celsius scales.

There are $100°$ (or units) on the Celsius scale from the boiling point to the freezing point of water. In the equivalent range on the Fahrenheit scale there are 180 units. To compare the two, one may use a ratio-proportion method, that is, $100°C$ is to $180°F$ as 1 is to X.

$$\frac{100}{180} = \frac{1}{X}$$
$$100X = 180$$

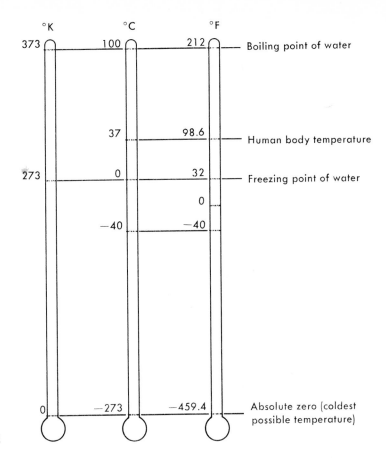

Fig. 5-1

Table 4

	Celsius	Fahrenheit
Boiling point	100°	212°
Freezing point	0°	32°
Number of degrees from boiling point to freezing point	100	180

$$X = 1.8 = 1\frac{4}{5} = \frac{9}{5}$$

Therefore, 1°C is equal to 1.8°F. Using common fractions, it can be seen that 1°C is equal to $^9/_5$°F. Similarly, 180°F is to 100°C as 1 is to X.

$$\frac{180}{100} = \frac{1}{X}$$

$$180X = 100$$

$$X = 0.556 = \frac{5}{9}$$

Therefore, 1°F is equal to 0.556°C, or 1°F is equal to $^5/_9$°C.

Notice that the comparison takes place only in a certain range (boiling point to

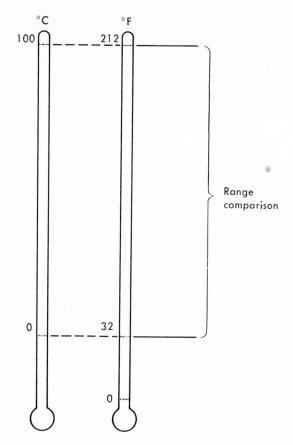

Fig. 5-2

freezing point of water), not from zero on both scales to a given point (Fig. 5-2). Since both scales were not compared from zero to a given point, this difference must be accounted for. The Fahrenheit scale has 32° more from the freezing point of water to the zero point.

TO CONVERT DEGREES CELSIUS TO DEGREES FAHRENHEIT

Since 1°C is equal to $^9/_5$° (or 1.8°) F, one must multiply the degrees Celsius readings by $^9/_5$ (or 1.8) to convert it to units of the magnitude of the Fahrenheit degree. This figure is then adjusted to the zero point of the Fahrenheit scale by the addition of 32 (see Fig. 5-2).

$$°F = \left(°C \times \frac{9}{5}\right) + 32$$

$$°F = (°C \times 1.8) + 32$$

EXAMPLE: Convert 37°C to °F.

$$°F = (°C \times 1.8) + 32$$
$$°F = (37 \times 1.8) + 32$$
$$°F = 66.6 + 32$$
$$°F = 98.6$$

TO CONVERT DEGREES FAHRENHEIT TO DEGREES CELSIUS

First adjust the zero point of the Fahrenheit scale to the zero point on the Celsius scale by subtracting 32 from the degree Fahrenheit value. Since 1°F is equal to $^5/_9$°C or 0.556°C, multiply the adjusted Fahrenheit value by $^5/_9$ (or 1.8) to get degrees Celsius.

$$°C = (°F - 32) \times \frac{5}{9}$$

$$°C = (°F - 32) \times 0.556$$

EXAMPLE: Convert 98.6°F to °C.

$$°C = (°F - 32) \times \frac{5}{9}$$

$$°C = (98.6 - 32) \times \frac{5}{9}$$

$$°C = 66.6 \times \frac{5}{9}$$

$$°C = 37$$

Another method that may be used to convert values between the Celsius and Fahrenheit scales is by use of the following formula:

$$\frac{°C}{°F - 32} = \frac{5}{9}$$

This formula can be derived using the following considerations. The freezing point of water is 0°C or 32°F. The range of temperature between the freezing and boiling point of water is 0°C to 100°C or 32°F to 212°F. Hence, 0°C = 32°F, and 100°C − 0°C = 212°F − 32°F. Therefore:

$$\frac{°C - 0}{°F - 32} = \frac{100 - 0}{212 - 32}$$

$$\frac{°C}{°F - 32} = \frac{100}{180}$$

$$\frac{°C}{°F - 32} = \frac{5}{9}$$

$$9 \times °C = 5 \times (°F - 32)$$
$$9 \times °C = 5 \times °F - 160$$

The simplified formula, 9C = 5F − 160, can be extracted from the preceding formula. This simple formula can be easily remembered and is useful for conversion in either direction between the Celsius and Fahrenheit scales.

EXAMPLE: Convert 37°C to °F.

$$9C = 5F - 160$$
$$9(37) = 5F - 160$$
$$333 = 5F - 160$$
$$5F = 333 + 160$$

$$F = \frac{493}{5}$$

$$F = 98.6$$

$$37°C = 98.6°F$$

EXAMPLE: Convert 98.6°F to °C.

$$9C = 5F - 160$$
$$9C = 5(98.6) - 160$$
$$C = \frac{493 - 160}{9}$$
$$C = \frac{333}{9}$$
$$C = 37$$
$$98.6°F = 37°C$$

Another simple means of converting between Fahrenheit and Celsius scales was offered by Martinek.* The temperature of $-40°$ is the same on the Celsius and the Fahrenheit scales. This conversion method and these equations for conversions between degrees Celsius and degrees Fahrenheit are based on the $9/5$ and $5/9$ relationships and the number 40. To convert degrees Fahrenheit to degrees Celsius, add 40 to the original temperature, multiply by $5/9$ and subtract 40 from this product. To convert degrees Celsius to degrees Fahrenheit, add 40 to the beginning temperature, multiply by $9/5$, and subtract 40 from the result.

REMEMBER:

$$[(°F + 40) \times 5/9)] -40 = °C$$
$$[(°C + 40) \times 9/5)] - 40 = °F$$

EXAMPLE: Convert 100°F to °C.

$$[(°F + 40) \times 5/9] - 40 = °C$$
$$[(100 + 40) \times 5/9] - 40 = °C$$
$$[140 \times 5/9] - 40 = °C$$
$$77.8 - 40 = °C$$
$$37.8 = °C$$

EXAMPLE: Convert 37°C to °F.

$$[(°C + 40) \times 9/5] - 40 = °F$$
$$[(37 + 40) \times 9/5] - 40 = °F$$
$$[77 \times 9/5] - 40 = °F$$
$$138.6 - 40 = °F$$
$$98.6 = °F$$

NOTE: If one is not sure which fraction to use, choose a familiar conversion point, such as 100°C = 212°F; it is obvious that to get from 100°C to 212°F one had to multiply by the larger fraction, $9/5$. Therefore, to convert degrees Celsius to degrees Fahrenheit, use $9/5$.

TO CONVERT DEGREES FAHRENHEIT TO DEGREES KELVIN

The simplest method to convert degrees Fahrenheit to degrees Kelvin is to first convert degrees Fahrenheit to degrees Celcius, and then add 273 to the result.

EXAMPLE: Convert 100°F to °K.

$$9C = 5F - 160$$
$$9C = 5(100) - 160$$
$$9C = 500 - 160$$
$$9C = 340$$
$$°C = 37.78$$

---

*Martinek, R. G.: Practical mathematics for the medical technologist, J. Am. Med. Tech. **34**:117-146, 1972.

$$°K = °C + 273$$
$$°K = 37.78 + 273$$
$$°K = 310.78$$

IN REVIEW: The following formulas have been presented. Use any of them; however, try to *understand* the underlying principle.

1. $°F = \left(°C \times \dfrac{9}{5}\right) + 32$

2. $°C = (°F - 32) \times \dfrac{5}{9}$

3. $\dfrac{°C}{°F - 32} = \dfrac{5}{9}$

4. $9C = 5F - 160$

5. $\left[(°F + 40) \times \dfrac{5}{9}\right] - 40 = °C$

6. $\left[(°C + 40) \times \dfrac{9}{5}\right] - 40 = °F$

Practice problems

Convert the following:

1. 25°C to °F
2. −20°C to °F
3. 260°C to °F

4. 150°F to °C
5. −20°F to °C
6. 400°F to °C

CHAPTER 6

Solutions

Solutions are mixtures of substances. The substances in a solution are not in chemical combination with one another, although chemical reactions can occur in solutions. However, the phases of solutions are not combined chemically one with another.

Most solutions can be thought of as having two parts or phases, the dispersed phase and the dispersing phase. The dispersed phase is the substance that is dissolved. This is often called the *solute*. The dispersing phase is the substance that dissolves the other. This material is called the *solvent*. In some solutions the distinction between the solvent and the solute becomes questionable. A one-to-one solution of alcohol in water is an example of such a solution. In such cases the worker will do well not to spend a great deal of mental energy trying to designate one as the solvent and the other as the solute.

Solutions found in biology and clinical systems are one of two types, *true* and *colloid*. In true solutions the particles of the solution are less than 1 nm in size. This is usually thought of as being dispersed at the atomic or molecular level. Colloidal solutions have solute particles that are between 1 and 200 nm in size. Such particles are usually considered to be aggregations of many molecules or atoms. One common exception to this in biology is the large molecules of nucleic acids, proteins, and the other macromolecules of protoplasm. These large molecules confer the properties of colloids on the mixture. Mixtures of materials in which the particles are larger than 200 nm are called *suspensions*. These mixtures will usually separate unless agitated. The true solutions and colloids will remain mixed without any agitation.

All substances will not form solutions with one another. Substances that *will* form solutions are said to be *miscible;* those that *will not* form solutions are said to be *immiscible* with one another. The degree of miscibility varies with environmental factors, such as temperature, pressure, and other dissolved materials.

When a solution contains the maximum amount of solute possible at a particular temperature and pressure, the solution is said to be *saturated*. Under some conditions a solution may contain more solute than the normal saturation amount. In such cases the solution is *supersaturated*. Such solutions will normally lose the excess solute easily.

Solutions are either uniform or are becoming uniform; that is, all parts of one solution contain equal proportions of all substances involved, or this situation is developing. This is due to the principle of diffusion. *Diffusion* is the physical principle that substances in solution have a tendency to move from regions of their greater concentration to regions of their lesser concentration. All substances in a solution diffuse at their own rates; that is, solvents and solutes diffuse through a solution.

In dealing with solutions, it soon becomes important to know or be able to measure the relative amounts of the substances in solution. This is referred to as concentration. Concentration may be measured in many ways. In all cases, concentration refers to the amount of one substance relative to the amounts of the other substances in the solution. Concentration values are not simply volumes or masses alone, but always exist in relation to volumes or masses of the other parts of the solution. In some methods of stating concentration values, the amount or proportion of one or more parts of the solution may not be stated but may be implied by the terminology of the concentration statement. Several methods of stating and manipulating concentration values are discussed in detail in this chapter.

PARTS

Often in the description of a procedure, the term *parts* is used. The use of this term allows the discussion of relationships in a procedure without being limited to any specific unit of measure. The important item being that this term is used to express a relationship; hence, the same unit of measure or multiple of the unit must be used throughout all of the related portions of a procedure. For example, if a procedure states, Mix one part of *A* with two parts of *B,* this can mean mix 1 gm of *A* with 2 gm of *B,* one ton of *A* with two tons of *B,* or 4 lb of *A* with 8 lb of *B.* Such expressions as one-to-one, 50-50, and two-to-three indicate situations in which the term *parts* is understood. The same considerations apply to such methods as apply to situations in which parts are used.

A unit of concentration frequently used in laboratory work is *parts per million* (ppm). This unit refers to a number of parts of one substance in 1 million parts of the solution. Hence, 5 ppm chlorine means that there are 5 gm chlorine in 1 million grams of water or that there are 5μg of chlorine in 1 gm water, as 1 gm equals 1 million micrograms.

The term *parts per billion* is used less frequently. This means so many parts of some substance in 1 billion parts of solution. In this situation any unit of measure may be used as long as the relationship is maintained.

BASIC WAYS OF MEASURING CONCENTRATION

Concentration can be measured in one of three basic ways: (1) weight per unit weight, (2) weight per unit volume, and (3) volume per unit volume. These are abbreviated w/w, w/v, and v/v, respectively.

The most accurate of the three ways is weight per unit weight, or w/w. In this system the property that is usually measured is not weight but mass. Technically, weight is the force of gravity pulling something toward Earth, whereas mass is the amount of matter in some object. The pound and its divisions are units of weight, whereas the gram and its multiples and divisions are units of mass. For all practical purposes, weight and mass can be used interchangeably, at least as long as the measurements are made on Earth. The term *weight* is traditionally used in the United States instead of the more proper term *mass*. The student of laboratory technology should recognize this situation. Concentration expressed as weight per unit weight is the most accurate method because the mass of a given amount of material does not vary with temperature or pressure as does the volume. Weight per unit weight concentration is almost always used for the measurement of solids in solid material. It is also used wherever extremely accurate and precise measurements are necessary.

A weight per unit volume (w/v) concentration is probably the most common value found in the biological laboratory. In this method a number of units of mass or weight are set relative to a given number of units of volume of solution. This system is most frequently used when the solute is a solid and the solvent is liquid. Molarity and normality are forms of weight per unit volume methods of stating concentration. The volume of a particular amount of material will vary with the temperature and, in the case of gases, pressure. The degree of variation is usually insufficient to significantly vary test results unless extremes of temperature variation are involved.

The last of the three methods of measuring concentration is volume per unit volume (v/v). The volume per unit volume method of concentration statement and preparation is almost always used when the solute and solvent are liquid. This method is the least accurate of the three. The variation of volume with temperature is found in both phases of the solution, but the degree of expansion and contraction varies with different substances. The advantage of this method is convenience. This becomes particularly important in work encountered in the clinical laboratory. The operator should consider how much latitude can be tolerated in making or testing solutions. If there is question as to whether or not the degree of variation is acceptable, some system of weight per unit weight or weight per unit volume should be used in the work.

Percent concentration

One of many ways used to express concentration is the method commonly called *percent concentration*. This method is used with all three of the basic comparisons of concentration statements, that is, w/w, w/v, and v/v. The consideration discussed for each type of comparison applies when each solution is used as a percent concentration.

The term *percent* is a shortened form of percentage and means parts per 100. This comes from the same root word as does the prefix *centi,* which is used in the metric system. Concentration values expressed in some manner to refer to parts per 100 are usually considered to be percent concentration values. Such concentration values usually involve the word percent or the symbol ''%.'' A few rather limited methods of expressing percent concentrations have been developed in the clinical laboratory. This does not preclude the correct use of other forms of such expression. However, the use of the established jargon of a particular laboratory decreases the possibility of confusion in communications.

Weight per unit weight (w/w). Percent concentration involving weight per unit weight is not used very much in the clinical or biological laboratory. This method of expressing concentration is the most accurate type of percent concentration; therefore, it is useful in the few incidences in which extraordinary precision is needed.

EXAMPLE: Make a 10%$^{w/w}$ NaCl aqueous solution.

To make this solution, mix 10 gm of NaCl with 90 gm H_2O. This makes a total of 100 gm of the 10%$^{w/w}$ salt solution. If more or less of the total solution is desired, then the mass of each of the constituent substances would have to be adjusted. Note that in a weight per unit weight solution any measurement must be in units of weight or mass.

EXAMPLE: Make 500 gm of a 10%$^{w/w}$ NaCl aqueous solution.

In this solution, 10%, by weight of the total, must be NaCl.

$$500 \text{ gm} \times 0.10 \ (10\%) = 50 \text{ gm}$$

Hence, to make 500 gm of this solution, one would mix 50 gm NaCl with 450 gm H_2O. The total result would be 500 gm, not milliliters, of 10%$^{w/w}$ NaCl in water.

Weight per unit volume (w/v). The weight per unit volume system of percent concentration is the most frequently used method in the clinical laboratory. This method is almost always used when a solid solute is mixed with a liquid solvent. It is also frequently used in solutions having a liquid solute in a liquid solvent. In the clinical laboratory and related situations, any time a weight per unit volume solution is described by a number followed by a percent symbol and there is nothing between the number and percent symbol (%), the concentration of the solution is expressed as *grams per 100 ml*. Consider a $10\%^{w/v}$ solution. This is a true percent expression in all respects if the solvent is water. Remember that 1 ml H_2O equals 1 gm H_2O under certain conditions; hence, 100 ml H_2O equals or is very nearly 100 gm H_2O. The system of grams per 100 ml is also used for other solvents even though 100 ml of other solvents does not equal 100 gm. In terms of weight per unit volume this remains a true percent value, although it is not parts per 100 in terms of weight per unit weight. This type of expression is sometimes written gm%.

Another expression of weight per unit volume percent concentration used in the clinical laboratory involves the use of fractional parts of the gram, but retains the unit volume of solution of 100 ml. Examples of this kind of expression are ''mg%'' and ''μg%.'' If mg% were a true weight per unit volume percent concentration, this would equal milligrams per 100 μl (since the microliter is the volume equivalent of the milligram), and μg% should equal micrograms per 100 ml. However, these are not expressions of percent concentration, but rather expressions of concentrations, which mean so many milligrams or micrograms of solute per 100 ml of solution. This is jargon. As most jargon expressions are likely to be confusing, the use of such terms should be avoided. However, they are used by many laboratory personnel, and any competent worker should understand their meaning. In an effort to correct this situation, the terms ''mg/dl'' and ''μg/dl'' have been proposed. One deciliter equals 100 ml, so milligram per deciliter is a true expression for what is meant by mg%. The relationship applies to microgram per deciliter and μg%.

Volume per unit volume (v/v). In most laboratory situations when a solution has a liquid solute in a liquid solvent, percent concentration is expressed as volume per unit volume (v/v). If a concentration value for a solution having both a liquid solute and solvent is expressed as % and there are no units of measure between the number and the percent sign, the value is assumed to be volume per unit volume.

EXAMPLE:

10% HCl = 10 ml concentration of HCl in 100 ml of solution

It is important to note that in the usual method for making a volume per unit volume solution and most weight per unit volume solutions, the desired amount of solute is placed in a vessel and enough solvent is added to make the desired total volume. The reason for this being that in some situations the volume of the solute plus the volume of solvent does not always equal the desired volume of the final solution.

This procedure is often referred to as *diluting up* the solute or *bringing up* the solution to some volume. The symbol ''$\uparrow$'' is used to mean this in working with solutions.

Frequently weight per unit volume procedures are used in making solutions having liquid solutes. In such cases the notation of the concentration value indicates weight per unit volume in some manner, such as $10\%^{w/v}$ HCl, 10 gm% HCl, or 10 mg/dl HCl.

CALCULATIONS INVOLVING CONCENTRATIONS

Problems involving concentrations are one of two types: (1) those in which the concentration values are not changed and (2) those in which the values are changed.

Problems not changing concentration

Most problems of this type involve variation in the amount of total solution. In working this type problem, one should fully understand the basis of a concentration value. In other words, the values in the comparison used in measuring concentration should be known and understood. In the forms of percent concentration notation commonly used in the clinical laboratory (w/v and v/v), the usual basis of the concentration is so many grams or milliliters of solute per 100 ml of solution. The most easily understood procedure to use in solving problems involving changes in solution volumes is the ratio-proportion procedure.

EXAMPLE: Make 300 ml of 5% NaCl.

Sodium chloride, NaCl, is a solid at the temperature at which this solution would be made; hence, this would be measured as w/v. A 5% NaCl solution would contain 5 gm NaCl per 100 ml of solution. The problem calls for 300 ml of solution. Set up a ratio and proportion using these data.

$$\frac{5 \text{ gm NaCl}}{100} = \frac{X}{300}$$

$$100X = 1500$$
$$X = 15 \text{ gm NaCl}$$

Therefore, 15 grams NaCl ↑ 300 ml will yield 300 ml of 5% NaCl.

EXAMPLE: A solution contains 24 gm of solute in 300 ml of solution. What is the percent concentration?

The problem states that there are 24 gm of solute per 300 ml of solution. Percent concentration is the number of grams of solute per 100 ml of solution. Arrange this information in a ratio-proportion setup.

$$\frac{24 \text{ gm}}{300 \text{ ml}} = \frac{X \text{ gm}}{100 \text{ ml}}$$

$$300X = 2400$$
$$X = 8$$

The solution has a concentration of 8%$^{w/v}$ solute.

EXAMPLE: How much of a 20% NaCl solution could be made from 50 gm NaCl?

A 20%$^{w/v}$ solution would contain 20 gm of solute per 100 ml of solution. The problem states that 50 gm of solute is to be used.

$$\frac{20 \text{ gm}}{100 \text{ ml}} = \frac{50 \text{ gm}}{X \text{ ml}}$$

$$20X \text{ ml} = 5000$$
$$X \text{ ml} = 250$$

Therefore, 50 grams of NaCl will make 250 ml of 20% NaCl.

In all these examples the concentration values have not been changed. The problems involved variations in the amount of solute or solution. Note that the procedures used in these examples did not involve formulas or precise methods. The available data were determined, the values to be calculated were established, and common sense was used in solving the problem. This is a much more useful method to use in solving most laboratory problems. The exclusive use of formulas limits the worker to those procedures for which a formula is known. If one must resort to a formula in solving some problem, then an attempt should be made to understand the mathematical relationships of the parts of the formula. For individuals lacking either sufficient intelligence or motivation, or both, to consider the preceding method, the following formulas may be useful in solving percent concentration problems in which the concentration remains unchanged.

1. To find an amount of solute to make a given amount of solution:

$$\frac{\% \times \text{Desired volume}}{100} = \text{Grams of solute to be diluted up to the desired volume}$$

2. To find the percent of a solution when the amount of solute and solution is known:

$$\frac{\text{Grams of solute} \times 100}{\text{Volume of solution}} = \text{Percent of solution}$$

Both of these formulas are modifications of the ratio-proportion procedure discussed previously. The basic ratio-proportion setup for this type problem consists of the following:

$$\frac{\text{Grams or milliliters of solute}}{100 \text{ ml of solution}} = \frac{\text{Grams or milliliters of solute}}{\text{Desired volume of solution}}$$

To work any problem of this type, one must know any three of the four values. If three values are known, the fourth can be calculated.

Problems changing concentration

In changing the concentration of a solution a basic relationship is used. This can be expressed as follows: the volume of one solution times the concentration of that solution equals the volume of a second solution times the concentration of the second solution. Expressed as a formula this relationship is as follows:

$$V_1 \times C_1 = V_2 \times C_2$$

Think about this relationship; try to understand why it is true. Also note that this is not a ratio-proportion relationship. The relationship between the volumes and concentrations involved in the two solutions is that of an *inverse* proportion; that is, when the volume of one solution is greater than the other, the concentration of the solution of greater volume is less. Careful study will show that the actual amount of one phase, either the solvent or the solute, will be equal in both solutions. The amount of the other phase will change from one solution to the other.

EXAMPLE: 20 ml of a 4% sugar solution will equal 40 ml of a 2% sugar solution.

Solution 1   Solution 2

$20 \times 4 = 40 \times 2$

The amount of sugar in both solutions is 0.8 gm, whereas the amount of water is changed.

As in ratio-proportion problems, three out of the four values of the formula must be known to solve for any one value.

The units of measure are the same for both solutions. If the volume of the first solution is measured in milliliters, the volume of the second solution will also be in milliliters. The form used to describe the concentration of one solution will be the same for the other solution.

$$\text{Milliters} \times \%^{w/w} = \text{Milliliters} \times \%^{w/w}$$
$$\text{Liters} \times \%^{w/v} = \text{Liters} \times \%^{w/v}$$

Any measure of volume may be used, as well as any system of concentration measure.

For example one may use liters, milliliters, barrels, or drams for volume and mole, $\%^{w/w}$, or milligrams per deciliter for concentration.

EXAMPLE: How much 30% alcohol is required to make 100 ml of 3%?

In solving such problems, first consider how to go about solving it. Notice that one concentration, 3%, is being made from another concentration, 30%. The concentration *changes;* therefore, the ratio-proportion method cannot be used. The $V_1 \times C_1 = V_2 \times C_2$ formula can be applied here. Fill in one side of the equation with the two pieces of information known about one solution; then, fill in the other side with the remaining information known about the other solution. In the preceding problem, the "100 ml of 3%" is a volume and concentration referring to the same solution, so these two factors go on one side of the equal sign. (In this type of problem, values of one solution are usually what is known or on hand; the values of the other solution are what is desired.)

$$\underbrace{V_1 \times C_1}_{\text{Solution 1}} = \underbrace{V_2 \times C_2}_{\text{Solution 2}}$$

$$100 \times 3 = V_2 \times C_2$$

Fill in the other side with the third piece of information, 30% (a concentration).

$$100 \times 3 = V_2 \times 30$$

This leaves the second volume as the unknown.

$$100 \times 3 = V_2 \times 30$$
$$V_2 \times 30 = 100 \times 3$$
$$30V_2 = 300$$
$$V_2 = 10$$

If 10 is put in the place of V_2, then

$$V_1 \times C_1 = V_2 \times C_2$$
$$100 \times 3 = V_2 \times 30$$
$$100 \times 3 = 10 \times 30$$
$$\text{Solution 1} = \text{Solution 2}$$

Therefore, 100 ml of 3% is equivalent to 10 ml of 30%, or if 10 ml of 30% is diluted up to 100 ml, the result would be 100 ml of 3% (10 ml of 30% ↑ 100 ml → 100 ml of 3%).

Knowing what an answer means and what to do with it is often the most difficult part of solving problems. For this reason write out answers in a complete form until the procedure becomes familiar. Understand *all* of the answer before proceeding.

EXAMPLE: 10 ml of 6% (solution 1) will make 100 ml of what percent?

$$V_1 \times C_1 = V_2 \times C_2$$
$$10 \times 6 = 100 \times C_2$$
$$100C_2 = 10 \times 6$$
$$100C_2 = 60$$
$$C_2 = 0.6$$

10 ml of 6% ↑ 100 ml → 100 ml of 0.6%

IN REVIEW: To use the formula, $V_1 \times C_1 = V_2 \times C_2$, the following factors must be considered:

1. The concentration must change (or be a different solution; a weaker solution is usually being made from a stronger one).
2. The concentration must be in the same units on both sides of the equation.
3. The two known pieces of information for one solution go on one side of the equation.
4. The other side is filled in appropriately, and the unknown is solved.

At times it becomes necessary to mix two or more solutions together. If two or more solutions are mixed together and one wants to know the concentration of the final solution, first, be sure all the concentrations are in the same units, then, use the $V_1 \times C_1 = V_2 \times C_2$ principle as follows:

$$(V_1 \times C_1) + (V_2 \times C_2) + (V_3 \times C_3) + \ldots = V_F \times C_F$$

Insert the volume and concentration of the solutions that were mixed in the $V_1 \times C_1$ and $V_2 \times C_2$ places. The V_F and C_F constitute the final volume (obtained by adding the volumes mixed together) and the final concentration (usually the unknown).

HYDRATES

Consideration of solutions involving hydrates is needed here. Some salts are available in several forms: in the anhydrous (no water) form and in the form of one or more hydrates. In a hydrate a number of water molecules are attached to each molecule of salt. If the salt comes in more than one hydration, the directions for preparing the solution should always specify the hydration intended. If this information is not given, assume the most common form to be the one required.

Often a prescribed hydrate of a salt is not readily available, but some other form is. One needs to be able to determine how much of the form available would be equivalent to the quantity of the form prescribed.

To do this, one must have a basis of comparison. The molecular weights of the substances involved may be used. Use a ratio-proportion setup to complete the problem.

EXAMPLE: A procedure states: Make a 10% solution of $CuSO_4$. Only $CuSo_4 \cdot H_2O$ is available.

$$10\% = 10 \text{ gm}/100 \text{ ml}$$

How much of the monohydrate would be equivalent to the 10 gm of the anhydrous form called for in the original procedure? The mol wt of $CuSO_4$ is 160, and the mol wt of $CuSO_4 \cdot H_2O$ is 178.

If 160 parts of the anhydrous form would equal 178 parts of the monohydrate

$$\frac{160 \text{ anhydrous}}{178 \text{ monohydrate}}$$

then 10 gm of the anhydrous would equal X gm of monohydrate.

$$\frac{160 \text{ anhydrous}}{178 \text{ monohydrate}} = \frac{10 \text{ anhydrous}}{X \text{ monohydrate}}$$

$$\frac{160}{178} = \frac{10}{X}$$

$$160X = 178 \times 10$$

$$160X = 1780$$

$$X = 11.125$$

If 11.125 gm of monohydrate were diluted up to 100 ml, the result would be 11.13% *monohydrate* $CuSO_4$ solution, but this would be equivalent to the 10% *anhydrous* $CuSO_4$ solution originally required. *Be sure this relationship is thoroughly understood before continuing.*

MOLARITY

In chemical reactions, atoms and molecules are either combined or separated during the reaction. In other words, chemical reactions take place at the level of the atoms and molecules of the reactants. A method that would allow the worker to know the relative number of reactant particles involved in a chemical reaction would be useful. The mole and the molarity measurement of concentration are such methods. A *mole* of a particular substance is the number of grams equal to the atomic or molecular weight of the substance. The atomic or molecular weight of a substance is the actual mass of the chemical particle (atom or molecule) relative to the mass of carbon. These values may be found in a handbook of chemistry and physics. Another method to determine the molecular weight of a compound is to add the atomic weights of the atoms comprising the molecule.

EXAMPLE: Find the molecular weight (mol wt) of NaCl.

$$\text{Atomic wt of Na} = 23$$
$$\text{Atomic wt of Cl} = \underline{35.5}$$
$$58.5$$

The atomic weight for sodium (Na) is 23; that for chlorine (Cl) is 35.5; hence, the molecular weight for sodium chloride is 58.5. One mole of sodium chloride equals 58.5 gm. The term *gram molecular weight* is often used as a definition of *mole*.

EXAMPLE: Find the mol wt of H_2SO_4.

$$2H = 1 \times 2 = 2$$
$$1S = 32 \times 1 = 32$$
$$4O = 16 \times 4 = \underline{64}$$
$$\text{mol wt of } H_2SO_4 = 98$$

Therefore, 1 gm mol wt of sulfuric acid equals 1 mole of sulfuric acid, which equals 98 gm.

One mole of any substance will contain approximately 6.02×10^{23} particles (Avogadro's number). A *1 molar solution* contains 1 mole of solute per liter of solution, that is, 1 mole of solute ↑ 1000 ml equal a 1 molar solution. The total volume is 1000 ml, since the solute is *diluted up to* 1 liter (l).

Molarity (M) is a number that expresses the number of moles of substance in 1 liter of solution. In solving molarity problems, there are two main procedures that are commonly used. The first procedure is based on the following basic formula:

$$\text{Molecular weight} \times \text{Molarity} = \text{Grams/Liter}$$

This formula is based on the fact that molarity is equal to the number of moles/liter; for example, a 2M solution contains 2 moles/l, and a 0.5M solution contains 0.5 moles/l.

The molecular weight of the substance times the molarity of the solution to be made will equal the number of grams of solute to dilute up to 1000 ml. This will make 1000 ml of the desired molarity.

Remember this relationship, for most of the formulas used to calculate values relating to molarity, molality, and normality will be modifications of it.

EXAMPLE: Make 1000 ml of 0.5M NaCl. The mol wt of NaCl is 58.5.

$$\text{mol wt} \times M = \text{gm/l}$$
$$58.5 \times 0.5 = 29.25 \text{ gm/l}$$
$$29.25 \text{ gm NaCl} \uparrow 1000 \text{ ml} \rightarrow 1000 \text{ ml of } 0.5M \text{ NaCl}$$

This formula may also be used to find the molarity of a solution. The formula expressed another way becomes the following:

$$\text{mol wt} \times M = \text{gm/l}$$

$$M = \frac{\text{gm/l}}{\text{mol wt}}$$

EXAMPLE: There are 300 gm NaCl per liter of solution. What is the molarity of the solution?

$$M = \frac{\text{gm/l}}{\text{mol wt}}$$

$$M = \frac{300}{58.5}$$

$$\text{Molarity} = 5.13$$

The concentration of this solution is 5.13M; that is, it contains 5.13 moles/l.

Another expression with which one should be familiar is *millimole* (mmole). A milligram molecular weight (that is, the molecular weight expressed in milligrams) is a millimole. In contrast to the molarity (or number of moles per liter), which is

$$\frac{\text{gm/l}}{\text{mol wt}}$$

the number of millimoles per liter is

$$\frac{\text{mg/l}}{\text{mol wt}}$$

A millimole is 1/1000 mole, and 1 mole equals 1000 mmoles.

To convert moles to millimoles, multiply the number of moles by 1000.

To convert millimoles to moles, divide the number of millimoles by 1000.

To retain the same concentration when making solutions involving millimoles of solute, divide the volume of the solution by 1000.

$$\text{Moles/Liter} = \text{Millimoles/Milliliter}$$
$$1\text{M} = 1 \text{ mole/l}$$
$$= 1000 \text{ mmole/l}$$
$$= 1000 \text{ mmole/1000 ml}$$
$$= \textcircled{1} \text{mmole/ml}$$
$$6\text{M} = 6 \text{ moles/l}$$
$$= 6000 \text{ mmole/l}$$
$$= 6000 \text{ mmole/1000 ml}$$
$$= \textcircled{6} \text{mmole/ml}$$

Therefore, if the number of millimoles/milliliters is known, the molarity is known automatically.

EXAMPLE: A solution contains 3.5 mmole/ml. What is the molarity of the solution?

This may be solved the long way by finding out the number of moles/l.
1. 3.5 mmole/ml would be 3500 mmole/1000 ml.
2. 3500 mmole/1000 ml would be 3.5 moles/1000 ml.
3. 3.5 moles/1000 ml is 3.5 moles/l.
4. The number of moles/l *is* the molarity; therefore, the molarity is 3.5.

On the other hand, one could simply look at the problem and remember that the number of millimoles per milliliter is numerically equal to the molarity, and the answer 3.5M would be evident.

IN REVIEW:

1. 1 gm mol wt = 1 mole
2. 1 mg mol wt = 1 mmole
3. 1 mole = 1000 mmole
4. mol wt × M = gm/l

$$\text{M} = \frac{\text{gm/l}}{\text{mol wt}}$$

5. M = mmole/ml

The second procedure that may be used involves the use of *ratio and proportion*. Unlike percent, molarity is always based on 1000. Remember that molarity is based on the number of grams per liter, so always work toward this relationship to help solve problems.

EXAMPLE: There are 20 gm NaCl in 400 ml of solution. What is its molarity?

To solve this problem, first, determine the number of grams per 1000 ml, as molarity equals the number of grams per liter divided by the molecular weight.

$$\text{M} = \frac{\text{gm/l}}{\text{mol wt}}$$

To find the number of grams in 1000 ml, use ratio and proportion. That is, 20 gm in 400 ml would be the same as X gm in 1000 ml.

$$20:400 = X:1000$$

$$\frac{20}{400} = \frac{X}{1000}$$

$$400X = 20,000$$
$$X = 50$$

There would be 50 gm in 1000 ml. Now that the number of grams in 1000 ml is known, fill in the following formula:

$$\text{M} = \frac{\text{gm/l}}{\text{mol wt}}$$

$$\text{M} = \frac{50}{58.5}$$

$$\text{M} = 0.85$$

The concentration of the solution is 0.85M.

EXAMPLE: Make 300 ml of 6M NaCl.

$$\text{mol wt} \times \text{M} = \text{gm/l}$$
$$58.5 \times 6 = 351 \text{ gm/l}$$

It would take 351 gm NaCl to make 1 liter of 6M solution. However, only 300 ml is to be made; therefore, 351 gm are to 1000 ml as X gm are to 300 ml.

$$351:1000 = X:300$$

$$\frac{351}{1000} = \frac{X}{300}$$

$$1000X = 105,300$$
$$X = 105.3 \text{ gm}$$

$$105.3 \text{ gm} \uparrow 300 \text{ ml} \rightarrow 300 \text{ ml of 6M NaCl}$$

IN REVIEW:

1. Molarity is always based on grams per 1000 ml of solution.
2. For any volume other than 1000 ml use a ratio-proportion procedure to determine the answer.

A combination of these two procedures, plus a little exercise in common sense, will usually solve most problems involving molarity.

MOLALITY

Molality is a system of expressing concentration and is similar to molarity. The molal concentration of a solution is equal to the number of *moles of solute per 1000 gm of solvent*. This is a mass per unit mass basis of measuring concentration. Because of this, molal concentration is independent of temperature variation. It is a more accurate method of measuring concentration than molarity. It is usually much less convenient than molarity and is infrequently used in the clinical or biological laboratory.

The volume of a given mass of a molal solution varies with temperature, the density of the materials used, and the pattern of the interaction of molecules of solutes and solvent. However, the relative masses of the constituents of the solution remain constant.

A 1 molal solution could be made by placing 1 mole (1 gm mol wt) in 1000 gm of solvent. This solution may have a volume greater or less than the volume of the separate parts of the mixture. No portion of the preparation of a molal solution uses volume as a method of measure.

OSMOLARITY

Still another measure of concentration is osmolarity. This value provides an estimate of the osmotic activity of the solution by indicating the relative number of particles dissolved in the solution. In general, the osmotic activity is more or less directly proportional to the number of free particles in a given amount of solution. In most biological fluids the charge of the particles does not greatly affect the osmotic potential. Hence, the concentration of separate particles in such solutions determines the osmotic activity.

One *osmole* of any substance is equal to 1 gm mol wt divided by the number of particles formed by the dissociation of the molecules. For those materials that do not ionize, 1 osmole is equal to 1 mole. For example, 1 osmole of glucose is equal to 1 mole of glucose (180 gm). Glucose does not dissociate in aqueous solutions. However, a molecule of sodium chloride will completely ionize in water. It will form one sodium and one chloride ion. One osmole of NaCl is equal to 1 gm mol wt divided by the number of particles formed upon dissociation. The molecular weight of NaCl is 58.5; hence

$$1 \text{ osmole NaCl} = \frac{58.5}{2} = 29.25 \text{ gm}$$

The osmolarity of any solution is dependent only on the number, not the nature, of particles in solution. The osmolarity of a solution of a given substance may be found by multiplying the molar concentration by the number of particles per mole resulting from ionization. Frequently the term *osmolality* is used. This is related to osmolarity in the same way that molality is related to molarity. Osmolarity measurements vary with temperature and are not as accurate as osmolality. However, at the concentration of the solutes of the body fluids there is little difference between the osmolality and the osmolarity of a solution, and the two are frequently used interchangeably.

Osmolarity (osmoles/l) = Molarity × Number of particles/Molecule resulting from ionization

This assumes 100% ionization, for the degree of ionization affects the osmolarity of a solution. However, the most common solutions for which osmolarity is determined are biological fluids. Since the concentration of electrolytes in these fluids is so low, complete dissociation is usually assumed.

Because of these low concentrations it is usually more convenient to measure osmolarity in terms of milliosmoles. One milliosmole (mOsmole) equals 1/1000 osmoles.

$$1 \text{ mOsmole} = \frac{1 \text{ mmole}}{\text{Particles/Molecule on dissociation}}$$

mOsmoles/l = mmoles/l × Particles/Molecule from ionization

EXAMPLE: A NaCl solution contains 50 mmoles/l; what is its concentration in mOsmoles/l?

$$mOsmoles/l = 50 \times 2$$
$$mOsmoles/l = 100$$

In physiologic fluids, such as plasma and urine, the osmotic activity is due to the combined osmotic activity of the substances that are dissolved in them. Therefore, to obtain the osmolarity, it would be necessary to calculate it from the concentration and degree of ionization of each constituent in the mixture. The osmolarity of such fluids is therefore most easily determined by measuring the *freezing-point depression.* The freezing point of water is depressed 1.86°C when solute is added to make a 1 osmolal (1 osmole/kg) solution; therefore, 1 osmole of any solute is that amount which will depress the freezing point of 1 kg of water by 1.86°C. One milliosmole of osmotic activity per liter is equivalent to the depression in the freezing point of a solution 0.00186°C below that of water (taken as 0°C); hence

$$1 \text{ osmole} = \Delta 1.86°C$$
$$1 \text{ mOsmole} = \Delta 0.00186°C$$

EXAMPLE: The freezing point of a sample of human plasma was found to be −0.62°C. What would be the milliosmolarity?

1 mOsmole gives $\Delta 0.00186$; therefore, X mOsmoles would give $\Delta 0.62$.

$$\frac{1}{0.00186} = \frac{X}{0.62}$$
$$0.00186X = 0.62$$
$$X = 333.3$$
$$\Delta 0.62 = 333.3 \text{ mOsmoles/l}$$

NORMALITY

If the mechanisms of molarity are understood, there should be no difficulty in understanding normality; normality and molarity are based on the same principles with one major change. Molarity is based on molecular weight (mol wt); normality is based on *equivalent weight* (eq wt). By definition, a gram equivalent weight of an element or compound is the mass that will combine with or replace 1 mole of hydrogen.

The materials used to make normal solutions dissociate or separate into positive or negative ions. Normality considers the ability of the ions to combine with other ions. For example, potassium hydroxide, KOH, dissociates into $1K^+$ ion and $1OH^-$ ion. Sulfuric acid, H_2SO_4, dissociates into $2H^+$ ions and $1SO_4^=$ ion. One mole of K^+ will replace 1 mole of H^+ in a chemical reaction; hence, KOH has an equivalent weight equal to 1 mole of KOH. Consider the combining ability of the sulfate ion, $SO_4^=$. One mole of this ion will combine with 2 moles of hydrogen. Since 1 gm eq wt of an element or compound is the mass that will combine with 1 mole of hydrogen, then 1 gm eq wt of H_2SO_4 equals 0.5 mole, because $2H^+$ ions will combine with $1SO_4$ ion. For purposes of this book, the gram equivalent weight of a compound or element may be considered to be equal to the gram molecular weight divided by the total positive valence of the constituent ions of the material considered.

One very common exception to this rule is that situation found in oxidation-reduction reactions. The calculations for this type of chemical reaction are performed rarely in the medical laboratory. For this reason, these reactions will not be considered in this book.

As a general rule, the equivalent weight of an element or compound is equal to the molecular weight divided by the valence. It should be clear from this rule that for monovalent ions the equivalent weight is equal to the molecular weight, but for polyvalent ions the equivalent weight becomes smaller than the molecular weight. Therefore, *equivalent weight is always equal to or less than molecular weight*. (This rule will be restated and used later in this chapter.)

One limitation to the normality system is that, depending on the reaction in which it is used, a given solution may have more than one normality because it may have more than one equivalent weight. However, the molarity of a solution is fixed, since there is only *one* molecular weight of any given substance.

Why then is normality considered more important in chemical reactions? Substances react together on the basis of an equal number of chemically active particles. Because equal weights of different substances contain a different number of chemically active particles, equal gram concentrations of elements or compounds cannot be indiscriminately added together. However, when gram units are converted to equivalents, the concentrations of elements or compounds are expressed in terms of their *combining weights;* that is, they may then be freely added together without regard to the nature of the substance, since 1 eq of any substance will always contain the same number of chemically active particles as 1 eq of any other substance, for example, 1 eq of Na = 1 eq H_2SO_4 = 1 eq $CaCl_2$. A 1 gm eq wt (the equivalent weight expressed in grams) equals 1 eq.

A 1 Normal (N) solution contains 1 gm eq (or 1 eq) of solute in 1000 ml of solution.

$$\text{1 gm eq wt} \uparrow \text{1000 ml} \rightarrow \text{1N solution}$$

Therefore, normality is a number that represents the *number* of equivalent weights (or equivalents) of solute in 1 liter of solution. A 1N solution = 1 eq/l, 6N = 6 eq/l, and 0.3N = 0.3 eq/l.

A term with which one should become familiar before proceeding is *milliequivalent* (mEq). This has the same relation to equivalent as millimole has to mole.

1. mg eq wt (the equivalent weight expressed in milligrams) = 1 mEq

2. $\dfrac{\text{mg}}{\text{eq wt}}$ = mEq

3. 1 eq = 1000 mEq

4. 1 mEq = $\dfrac{1}{1000}$ eq

The two procedures usually used for solving normality problems are the same as those used for solving molarity, except the equivalent weight is used in the formula instead of the molecular weight.

Formula use

Molarity (M)	Normality (N)
mol wt × M = gm/l	eq wt × N = gm/l

The equivalent weight for the substance times the desired normality equals the number of grams of solute to dilute with enough distilled water to make 1 liter of solution with the desired normality. If any two of the values are known, solve for the third.

EXAMPLE: Make 6N NaCl.

$$\text{mol wt} = 58.5$$
$$\text{eq wt} = 58.5$$

$$\text{eq wt} \times \text{N} = \text{gm/l}$$
$$58.5 \times 6 = 351.0 \text{ gm/l}$$

$$351.0 \text{ gm NaCl} \uparrow 1000 \text{ ml} \rightarrow 1 \text{ liter of 6N NaCl}$$

EXAMPLE: What is the normality of a NaOH solution containing 200 gm NaOH/l?

$$\text{eq wt} \times \text{N} = \text{gm/l}$$

$$\text{N} = \frac{\text{gm/l}}{\text{eq wt}}$$

$$\text{N} = \frac{200}{40}$$

$$\text{N} = 5$$

As with molarity, an easy way to find normality is to remember that the number of mEq/ml is numerically equal to normality.

$$
\begin{aligned}
1\text{N} &= 1 \text{ eq/l} \\
&= 1000 \text{ mEq/l} \\
&= 1000 \text{ mEq/1000 ml} \\
&= \enclose{circle}{1} \text{ mEq/ml}
\end{aligned}
$$

$$
\begin{aligned}
0.3\text{N} &= 0.3 \text{ eq/l} \\
&= 300 \text{ mEq/l} \\
&= 300 \text{ mEq/1000 ml} \\
&= \enclose{circle}{0.3} \text{ mEq/ml}
\end{aligned}
$$

IN REVIEW:

1. 1 gm eq wt = 1 eq
2. 1 mg eq wt = 1 mEq
3. 1 eq = 1000 mEq
4. Normality of a solution is a number expressing the number of equivalents per liter
5. eq wt = $\dfrac{\text{mol wt}}{\text{Valence}}$
6. Equivalent weight is always equal to or less than molecular weight
7. The number of milliequivalents per milliliter is numerically equal to the normality
8. 1 eq of any substance = 1 eq of any other substance
9. 1 mEq of any substance = 1 mEq of any other substance

Ratio-proportion setup

As molarity, normality is based on grams per 1000 ml.

$$\text{eq wt} \times \text{N} = \text{gm/l}$$

First determine this figure (gm/l), then complete the solution.

EXAMPLE: Make 300 ml of a 0.4N NaOH solution.

$$\text{mol wt} = 40$$
$$\text{eq wt} = 40$$
$$\text{eq wt} \times \text{N} = \text{gm/l}$$
$$40 \times 0.4 = 16.0 \text{ gm/l}$$

It would take 16 gm NaOH to make 1 liter of solution. However, only 300 ml is required; therefore, use ratio and proportion as follows: 16 is to 1000 as X is to 300.

$$\frac{16}{1000} = \frac{X}{300}$$

$$1000X = 4800$$
$$X = 4.8$$

Therefore, 4.8 gm NaOH ↑ 300 ml → 300 ml of a 0.4N solution of NaOH.

EXAMPLE: There are 80 gm NaOH in 400 ml of solution. What is the normality?

Eighty grams are to 400 ml as X gm are to 1000 ml.

$$\frac{80}{400} = \frac{X}{1000}$$

$$400X = 80,000$$
$$X = 200 \text{ gm/l}$$

$$N = \frac{\text{gm/l}}{\text{eq wt}}$$

$$N = \frac{200}{40}$$

$$N = 5$$

$V_1 \times C_1 = V_2 \times C_2$ using normality

As stated earlier, when using $V_1 \times C_1 = V_2 \times C_2$, one may state the concentration in %, M, or N. When the two concentrations are in different units, it is necessary to change one unit to match the other. It usually does not matter which unit is changed as long as the units are the same. However, there is one exception. If the problem states: *neutralize, react with,* or *equal,* then both the units must be in normality, because only in normality does 1 ml of a given normality equal 1 ml of the same normality in another substance. (Recall that 1 eq of an substance equals 1 eq of any other substance and that normality is the number of equivalents per liter.)

IN REVIEW:

1. Normality is always based on gm/1000 ml of solution.
2. For any volume other than 1000 ml, use a ratio-proportion setup to determine the answer.

Perhaps a word should be said about the different ways that normality and molarity may be written or expressed when the normality and molarity are fractions with the numeral 1 as the numerator. A solution with a normality of $^1/_{10}$ may be written $^1/_{10}$N, 0.1N, or N/10 (the N taking the place of the 1 in the numerator). $^1/_5$N may be expressed $^1/_5$N, 0.2N, or N/5.

SPECIFIC GRAVITY

Specific gravity is a method of measuring density. Density is the amount of matter in a given volume. In other words, density is the mass per unit volume. Specific gravity is a ratio between the mass of a substance and the mass of an equal volume of pure water at 4°C.

$$\text{Specific gravity} = \frac{\text{Weight of solid or liquid}}{\text{Weight of equal volume of water at 4°C}}$$

Since 1 ml of water has a mass of 1 gm, specific gravity is equal to the mass in grams of 1 ml of any substance. Materials less dense than water have a specific gravity of less than one, whereas materials more dense than water have a specific gravity greater than one.

The most frequent use of specific gravity values in the clinical laboratory is in working with concentrated commercial liquids. Often a bottle label will show the specific gravity and a value called either *assay* or *percent purity*. These values indicate the mass of 1 ml of the solution and the proportion of the solution by weight that is the substance desired. Using these values, one can determine the actual amount of the substance in a given volume of the supply solution.

EXAMPLE: The values listed on the label of a bottle of nitric acid are specific gravity (sp gr) 1.42 and assay 70%. What do these values mean?

These values mean that 1 ml of the solution has the mass of 1.42 gm and that 70% of this mass is HNO_3.

To find how much HNO_3 is in 1 ml of the supply solution, multiply the specific gravity by the assay percent. The answer is the number of grams of HNO_3 per milliliter of the solution.

$$\begin{array}{ll} 1.42 & \text{sp gr of solution} \\ \underline{0.70} & \text{\% } HNO_3 \\ 0.9940 \end{array}$$

Hence, there are 0.994 gm HNO_3 per milliliter of solution. This information is used in making other solutions from concentrated solutions.

EXAMPLE: Make 1 liter of 10%$^{w/v}$ HNO_3 solution. Use the information from the preceding example (a nitric acid supply having a specific gravity of 1.42 and an assay of 70%; hence a supply solution containing 0.994 gm of nitric acid per milliliter).

The instructions call for 1 liter (or 1000 ml) of a 10%$^{w/v}$ HNO_3 solution. The solution should contain 10 gm HNO_3 per 100 ml of solution. Find how much nitric acid would be in 1000 ml of this solution by using ratio and proportion.

$$\frac{10 \text{ gm}}{100 \text{ ml}} = \frac{X \text{ gm}}{1000 \text{ ml}}$$

$$100X = 1000$$
$$X = 100$$

One liter of 10%$^{w/v}$ HNO_3 solution will contain 100 gm.

The next part of the problem is to determine how much of the supply solution will contain 100 gm of nitric acid. Since each milliliter of the solution contains 0.994 gm of HNO_3, a ratio-proportion setup can be used to determine the volume of the supply solution containing 100 gm of HNO_3.

$$\frac{0.994 \text{ gm}}{1.0 \text{ ml}} = \frac{100 \text{ gm}}{X \text{ ml}}$$

$$0.994X = 100$$
$$X = 100.6 \text{ ml}$$

Therefore, 100 gm of pure nitric acid would be contained in 100.6 ml of solution. This 100.6 ml of the concentrated HNO_3 ↑ 1000 ml would give a 10.06%$^{v/v}$ solution of the supply solution that would also be in the 10%$^{w/v}$ HNO_3 solution called for in the problem.

This is not actually a weight per unit volume solution, since the nitric acid was not measured by weight but by volume. However, because water and solutions of water vary little in volume at the temperatures of the laboratory, the use of volume does not produce a degree of variation great enough to warrant the inconvenience of weighing highly corrosive liquids.

Two more examples of this type problem are given showing a greater variation in the values.

EXAMPLE: Make 250 ml of a 20%$^{w/v}$ HCl solution. The supply of concentrated HCl has a specific gravity of 1.19 and an assay of 38%. Find the amount of HCl per milliliter of supply solution.

$$1.19 \text{ sp gr}$$
$$\underline{0.38} \ \% \text{ assay}$$
$$952$$
$$\underline{357}$$
$$0.4522$$

There are 0.4522 gm HCl per milliliter of solution.

Next, determine how much HCl would be needed to produce 250 ml of a 20%$^{w/v}$ solution using ration and proportion.

$$\frac{20 \text{ gm}}{100 \text{ ml}} = \frac{X \text{ gm}}{250 \text{ ml}}$$
$$100X = 5000$$
$$X = 50$$

Therefore, 50 gm of HCl is needed in 250 ml of 20%$^{w/v}$ solution of HCl.

Now, how much supply solution is needed to yield 50 gm of the desired solution?

$$\frac{0.4522 \text{ gm}}{1 \text{ ml}} = \frac{50 \text{ gm}}{X \text{ ml}}$$
$$0.4522X = 50$$
$$X = 110.6 \text{ ml}$$

Therefore, 110.6 ml of the supply solution contains 50 gm HCl.

From the preceding calculations it is known that 110.6 ml of the supply solution diluted up to 250 ml will give a 20%$^{w/v}$ solution; remember that the *weight* was based on a volume measure. This would also be a 44.24%$^{v/v}$ solution of the supply solution. Try to calculate this.

EXAMPLE: Make a 0.5N HCl solution using the preceding supply of concentrated HCl.

To make a normal solution, the equivalent weight of the solute has to be known. In the case of HCl the equivalent weight equals 1 mole. The molecular weight of HCl is 36.5; hence, 1 mole of HCl equals 36.5 gm and 1 eq wt would equal 36.5 gm. A 1N solution would have the concentration of 1 eq wt/1 of solution. In this case 36.5 gm HCl/l would be a 1N solution, and 1 liter of a 0.5N HCl solution would contain one-half of a 1N solution.

$$\text{eq wt} \times \text{N} = \text{gm/l}$$
$$36.5 \times 0.5 = 18.25 \text{ gm/l}$$

How much of the supply solution of HCl would contain 18.25 gm? From calculations in the last problem, it was determined that the supply solution contained 0.4522 gm HCl/ml. To determine how much solution is needed to contain 18.25 gm of HCl, use a ratio-proportion setup.

$$\frac{0.4522 \text{ gm}}{1 \text{ ml}} = \frac{18.25 \text{ gm}}{X \text{ ml}}$$
$$0.4522X = 40.4 \text{ ml}$$

Hence, 40.4 ml supply solution ↑ 1000 ml equals a 0.5N HCl solution.

CONCENTRATION RELATIONSHIPS

There are several instances in which the form a concentration value is expressed is not the form desired. Consider the following examples:

1. A procedure may call for 0.5M NaOH, and all that is on hand is 10% NaOH.
2. A problem may ask how much 5M HCl would be neutralized by a certain amount of 10N NaOH.
3. An answer in a given test procedure may be in mg/dl, and the physician wants it in mEq/l.

The relationship between these various units and how to convert them should present no problem to the worker, if this individual understands the material covered in this chapter.

This discussion concerns some methods to use in converting one type of concentration to another.

Consider the conversion of percent to molarity or normality. Remember two basic facts: (1) percent, unless stated otherwise, is grams per 100 ml and (2) molarity and normality are based on grams per liter.

Recall the basic molarity and normality formulas:

$$\text{mol wt} \times M = \text{gm/l} \qquad\qquad \text{eq wt} \times N = \text{gm/l}$$

$$M = \frac{\text{gm/l}}{\text{mol wt}} \qquad\qquad N = \frac{\text{gm/l}}{\text{eq wt}}$$

If the grams per liter and the molecular or equivalent weights are known, one can find molarity and normality. The percent equals the number of grams per 100 ml; therefore, multiply the percent by ten to get the number of grams per liter. One point about percent needs to be brought out here. Since molarity and normality are based on grams (weight) per liter, the percent used in these formulas *must* be a weight per unit volume concentration (gm/100 ml). A volume per unit volume concentration *cannot* be used unless it is first converted to a weight per unit volume concentration. Consider a 10% NaCl solution. This solution contains 10 gm of NaCl per 100 ml of solution. Multiply the 10 gm in 100 ml by ten to get the number of grams in 1000 ml ($10 \times 10 = 100$ gm/1000 ml). Using this information, one may derive the formula for converting percent to molarity or normality, or vice versa.

$$\text{mol wt} \times M = \text{gm/l} \qquad\qquad \text{eq wt} \times N = \text{gm/l}$$

$$M = \frac{\text{gm/l}}{\text{mol wt}} \qquad\qquad N = \frac{\text{gm/l}}{\text{eq wt}}$$

$$M = \frac{\text{gm/100 ml} \times 10}{\text{mol wt}} \qquad\qquad N = \frac{\text{gm/100 ml} \times 10}{\text{eq wt}}$$

$$M = \frac{\% \times 10}{\text{mol wt}} \qquad\qquad N = \frac{\% \times 10}{\text{eq wt}}$$

The only difference between converting percent to molarity or normality is the use of molecular weight for molarity and equivalent weight for normality.

These formulas may be used to convert from percent to molarity or normality or to convert from molarity and normality to percent. Fill in all known quantities and solve for X. There is no need to memorize them. If one remembers the basic formula (mol wt $\times M = $ gm/l) and understands it, the conversion formula can be figured out when it is needed.

EXAMPLE: Convert 30% NaCl to molarity.

$$M = \frac{\% \times 10}{\text{mole wt}}$$

$$M = \frac{30 \times 10}{58.5}$$

$$M = \frac{300}{58.6}$$

$$M = 5.13$$

$$30\% \text{ NaCl} = 5.13\text{M NaCl}$$

EXAMPLE: Convert 6M NaOH to percent.

$$\text{M} = \frac{\% \times 10}{\text{mol wt}}$$

$$6 = \frac{\% \times 10}{40}$$

$$6 \times 40 = \% \times 10$$
$$\% \times 10 = 240$$
$$\% = 24$$
$$6\text{N NaOH} = 24\%^{\text{w/v}} \text{ NaOH}$$

EXAMPLE: Convert 3N H_2SO_4 to percent.

$$\text{mol wt of } H_2SO_4 = 98$$
$$\text{eq wt of } H_2SO_4 = 49$$

$$\text{N} = \frac{\% \times 10}{\text{eq wt}}$$

$$3 = \frac{\% \times 10}{49}$$

$$3 \times 49 = \% \times 10$$
$$\% \times 10 = 147$$
$$\% = 14.7$$

$$3\text{N } H_2SO_4 = 14.7\%^{\text{w/v}}$$

Another type of conversion problem involves the conversion of milligrams per deciliter to milliequivalent per liter, or vice versa.

REMEMBER:

$$\text{eq wt} \times \text{N} = \text{gm/l}$$

$$\text{N(or eq/l)} = \frac{\text{gm/l}}{\text{eq wt}}$$

$$\text{mEq/l} = \frac{\text{mg/l}}{\text{eq wt}}$$

Recall that mg/dl means mg/100 ml; as in percent, multiply the number of mg/100 ml by ten to get the number of mg/1000 ml. Therefore

$$\text{mEq/l} = \frac{\text{mg/l}}{\text{eq wt}}$$

$$\text{mEq/l} = \frac{\text{mg/100 ml} \times 10}{\text{eq wt}}$$

$$\text{mEq/l} = \frac{\text{mg/dl} \times 10}{\text{eq wt}}$$

EXAMPLE: Express 300 mg/dl Cl as mEq/l Cl.

$$\text{mEq/l} = \frac{300 \times 10}{35.5}$$

$$\text{mEq/l} = \frac{3000}{35.5}$$

$$\text{mEq/l} = 84.51$$

$$300 \text{ mg/dl Cl} = 84.51 \text{ mEq/l Cl}$$

EXAMPLE: Express 150 mEq/l NaCl and mg/dl NaCl.

$$mEq/l = \frac{mg/dl \times 10}{eq\ wt}$$

$$150 = \frac{mg/dl \times 10}{58.5}$$

$$mg/dl \times 10 = 150 \times 58.5$$
$$mg/dl \times 10 = 8775$$
$$mg/dl = 877.5$$

$$150\ mEq/l\ NaCl = 877.5\ mg/dl\ NaCl$$

Notice that Cl has been converted to Cl and NaCl to NaCl. Suppose one were asked not only to change concentration units, but to change the values to the concentration of another substance as well.

EXAMPLE: Express 700 mg/dl NaCl as mEq/l Cl.

There are two main ways to go about solving this problem; use whichever makes the most sense.

1. First change mg/dl NaCl to mg/dl Cl by ratio and proportion using the molecular weights; then, convert mg/dl Cl to mEq/l Cl.

2. Recall that 1 mEq of any substance equals 1 mEq of any other substance; therefore, the number of mEq/l NaCl equals the number of mEq/l of Cl.

Compare the above problem worked both ways

$$\frac{35.5}{58.5} = \frac{X}{700}$$

$$58.5X = 700 \times 35.5$$
$$58.5X = 24,850$$
$$X = 424.8$$
$$700\ mg/dl\ NaCl = 424.8\ mg/dl\ Cl$$

$$mEq/l\ Cl = \frac{424.8 \times 10}{35.5}$$

$$mEq/l = \frac{4248}{35.5}$$

$$mEq/l = 119.66$$

$$424.9\ mg/dl\ Cl = 199.66\ mEq/l\ Cl$$

$$mEq/v\ NaCl = \frac{mg/dl \times 10}{eq\ wt}$$

$$mEq/l\ NaCl = \frac{700 \times 10}{58.5}$$

$$mEq/l\ NaCl = \frac{7000}{58.5}$$

$$mEq/l\ NaCl = 119.66$$

$$119.66\ mEq/l\ NaCl = 199.66\ mEq/l\ Cl$$

The preceding is true because of the relationship between the two. In the first method 700 mg/dl NaCl = 424.8 mg/dl Cl. If these two figures are converted to mEq/l the result is the following:

$$mEq/l\ NaCl = \frac{700 \times 10}{58.5}$$

$$mEq/l\ NaCl = 119.66$$

$$mEq/l\ Cl = \frac{424.8 \times 10}{35.5}$$

$$mEq/l\ Cl = 199.66$$

When converting mg/dl NaCl to mEq/l, use the eq wt of NaCl (58.5), and when converting mg/dl Cl to mEq/l use the eq wt of Cl (35.5).

Do the same problem in reverse
Convert 119.66 mEq/l Cl to mg/dl NaCl

Convert 119.66 mEq/l Cl to mg/dl Cl and then ratio-proportion mg/dl Cl to mg/dl NaCl.

$$119.66 = \frac{X \times 10}{35.5}$$

$$10X = 119.66 \times 35.5$$
$$10X = 4247.9$$
$$X = 424.8 \text{ mg/dl Cl}$$

$$\frac{35.5}{58.5} = \frac{424.8}{X}$$

$$35.5X = 58.5 \times 424.8$$
$$35.5X = 24,850.8$$
$$X = 700 \text{ mg/dl NaCl}$$

424.8 mg/dl Cl = 700 mg/dl NaCl
119.66 mEq/l Cl = 700 mg/dl NaCl

The 119.66 mEq/l Cl is also equal to 119.66 mEq/l NaCl, so convert 119.66 mEq/l NaCl to mg/dl NaCl.

$$119.66 = \frac{X \times 10}{58.5}$$

$$10X = 119.66 \times 58.5$$
$$10X = 7000.1$$
$$X = 700 \text{ mg/dl NaCl}$$

119.66 mEq/l Cl = 700 mg/dl NaCl

REMEMBER:

1. 1 mEq of any substance equals 1 mEq of any other substance.
2. To change one substance to equivalent milligrams another substance, use *ratio and proportion* and *milligrams* (not milliequivalent).

One should now be able to convert %$^{w/v}$ to molarity and normality and vice versa and mEq/l to mg% and vice versa. That only leaves one important category to consider —how to convert molarity to normality and normality to molarity.

The following are the formulas for these conversions:

$$N = M \times \text{Valence}$$

$$M = \frac{N}{\text{Valence}}$$

Recall that the normality of a solution must always equal or be greater than the molarity of the same solution. The reason being that normality is based on equivalent weight and molarity is based on molecular weight. To arrive at the equivalent weight, divide the molecular weight by the valence; therefore, the equivalent weight is always equal to or less than the molecular weight.

$$H_2SO_4 - \text{mol wt} = 98$$

$$\text{eq wt} = \frac{98}{2} = 49$$

A molecular weight may contain two or more equivalent weights. If this is the case and if a solution contained one molecular weight, it would contain two or more equivalent weights, and since molarity is the number of moles (molecular weight) per liter and normality is the number of equivalents (equivalent weights per liter), the molarity of that solution would be one and the normality would be two or more.

$$98 = 1 \text{ mol wt} = 1\text{M}$$
$$98 = 2 \text{ eq wt} = 2\text{N}$$

EXAMPLE: Convert 6N NaOH to molarity.
The valence of NaOH is one; therefore, the normality and the molarity are the same.

$$M = \frac{N}{\text{Valence}}$$

$$M = \frac{6}{1}$$

$$M = 6$$

$$6N\ NaOH = 6M\ NaOH$$

EXAMPLE: Convert $10M\ H_2SO_4$ to normality.

$$N = M \times Valence$$
$$N = 10 \times 2$$
$$N = 20$$
$$10M\ H_2SO_4 = 20N\ H_2SO_4$$

EXAMPLE: Express $0.6N\ H_3PO_4$ as molarity.

$$M = \frac{N}{Valence}$$

$$M = \frac{0.6}{3}$$

$$M = 0.2$$
$$0.6N\ H_3PO_4 = 0.2M\ H_3PO_4$$

Notice that in each case the normality is equal to or greater than the molarity.

IN REVIEW:

1. $M = \dfrac{\% \times 10}{mol\ wt}$

2. $N = \dfrac{\% \times 10}{eq\ wt}$

3. $mEq/l = \dfrac{mg\% \times 10}{eq\ wt}$

4. $N = M \times Valence$

5. $M = \dfrac{N}{Valence}$

Conversion of volume percent CO_2 to millimoles per liter

A rather specialized concentration conversion is the changing of the concentration expression of carbon dioxide from milliliters per 100 ml of serum to millimoles per liter.

Under standard conditions of temperature and pressure, 1 mole (1000 mmoles) of a perfect gas occipies 22.4 l of space. However, carbon dioxide is not a perfect gas. One mole of this gas occupies 22.260 l (22,260 ml) under standard conditions. Carbon dioxide determinations are frequently reported as volume percent (ml/100 ml of serum). Many people prefer to have the CO_2 concentration in millimoles per liter. Since 1000 mmoles CO_2 occupies 22,260 ml of space, 22.26 ml CO_2 equals 1 mmole. Thus, the number of milliliters of CO_2 divided by 22.26 will give the number of millimoles.

The number of milliliters of CO_2 per 100 ml serum can be converted to the number of millimoles per liter in the following manner:

$$vol\% = ml\ CO_2/100\ ml\ serum$$

$$\frac{vol\%}{22.26} = mmoles/100\ ml$$

$$\frac{vol\% \times 10}{22.26} = mmoles/l$$

$$\frac{vol\%}{2.226} = mmoles/l$$

or

$$vol\% \times \frac{1}{2.226} = mmoles/l$$

Thus, to convert vol% to mmoles/l:

$$vol\% \times 0.45 = mmoles/l$$

Recall

$$\frac{vol\%}{2.226} = mmoles/l$$

Thus, to convert mmoles/l to vol%:

$$vol\% = mmoles/l \times 2.226$$

Practice problems

Percent

1. Make 100 ml of 6% NaCl from 10%.
2. 30 ml of 9% can be made from how much 10%?
3. How would one make 2000 ml of 30% HCl?
4. 150 ml of 0.2% can be made from 3 ml of what percent?
5. How much NaCl is actually present in 5 ml of 20% NaCl?
6. How much 20% alcohol can be made from 30 ml of 5%?
7. How much 4% H_2SO_4 would be required to make 1000 ml of 0.5%?
8. Make 2000 ml of 30% NaCl.
9. How much 20% can be made from 1.5 ml of 70%?
10. There are 25 gm in 300 ml of solution. What is its percent concentration?
11. How much 20% solution can be made from 50 gm NaCl?

Hydrates

12. 500 ml of a 10% Na_2SO_4 · 10 H_2O solution is needed. Carry out the steps involved in making the required 10% solution using Na_2SO_4.
13. $CaCl_2$ is available; the procedure calls for a 5% $CaCl_2$ · 10 H_2O solution. What would be the procedure for making 3000 ml of the desired concentration?

Molarity

14. What weight of NaOH would be required to prepare 3000 ml of a 1.5M solution?
15. A solution contains 300 gm NaCl/l. What is its molarity?
16. There are 160 gm of H_2SO_4 in 400 ml of solution. What is the molarity of the solution?
17. 30 ml of 3M will make 240 ml of what molar?
18. How much 4M NaOH solution can be made with 40 gm NaOH?
19. In a solution of NaCl containing 300 mmoles in 250 ml of solution, what is the molarity?
20. If one has a 20 gm/400 ml solution that is 10M, what is the molecular weight of the substance?
21. To make a solution of $CaCl_2$ that contains 1/10 gm mole/l, how much $CaCl_2$ would be needed?
22. How many grams of NaOH are present in 200 ml of a 6M solution of sodium hydroxide?
23. How much sodium hydroxide would be present in 0.0078M aqueous KOH?
24. How much 0.01M can be made from 10 ml of 6M HCl?

Osmolarity

25. A solution contains 5 moles/l of a substance that yields 2 ions upon dissociation. What is its concentration in osmoles/l?

26. A solution of a substance that does not ionize has a concentration of 50 mmoles/l What is its concentration in mOsmoles/1?

27. A NaCl solution contains 720 mg NaCl/100 ml of solution. What is its concentration in mOsmoles/l?

28. A urine sample has a freezing point of $-0.71°$ C. What is its concentration in mOsmoles/l?

29. A solution contains 50 mOsmoles/l of NaCl and 150 mOsmoles/l of glucose. What would be its freezing point?

30. A solution of NaCl and glucose give a freezing point of $-0.92°$ C. It contains 150 mOsmoles/l of glucose. Give the concentration of NaCl in mOsmoles/l and molarity.

Normality

31. Make 500 ml of 6N H_3PO_4.

32. A 5N $CaCl_2$ · 10 H_2O solution is needed. $CaCl_2$ is available. How would one make the needed solution?

33. Given: 5 l of approximately 0.5N HCl. Wanted: exactly 0.5N HCl. When titrated, the solution was found to be 0.6N. How much water should be added to make the 0.5N solution desired?

34. What would be the normality of 40 gm of NaOH in 400 ml of solution?

35. How much 6N HCl will be required to neutralize 60 ml of 0.6N NaOH?

36. 8 ml of N/10 solution may be converted to N/100 solution by adding water to make a total of how many milliliters?

37. Make 2000 ml of N/6 HCl.

38. In a titration procedure, 20 ml of 2N solution were required to titrate 5 ml of an unknown solution. What is the normality of the unknown solution?

39. How many grams of NaCl will be in 200 ml of a 10N solution?

40. How would one make 3 l of 3N H_3PO_4?

41. How many milliequivalents of $Ba(OH)_2$ are there in 200 ml of 0.1N $Ba(OH)_2$?

42. Make 200 ml of N/4 $BaCl_2$.

43. There are 20 mEq in 200 ml of a NaOH solution. What is the normality?

44. How would one prepare 250 ml of 0.04N $BaSO_4$?

45. How many milliliters of a 5N solution can be made from 50 gm $CaCl_2$?

46. 300 ml of a 2N $CaCl_2$ solution is desired. $CaCl_2$ · 10 H_2O is on hand. How should one proceed?

47. Make 1500 ml of 3N H_2SO_4.

48. A procedure calls for 6N $AgNO_3$. 5 ml is used for each test. Six tests and three controls per day, seven days a week, are averaged. The solution is stable for three months. Pure $AgNO_3$ is ordered in 1 lb jars. It costs 20 cents per ounce. How much should be ordered for a six-month supply, and how much would it cost?

49. There are 300 mEq in 30 ml of an NaOH solution. What is its normality?

50. If 30 ml of 4N NaOH and 100 ml of 0.8N NaOH are mixed together, what would be the normality of the resulting solution?

51. How many milliliters of 6N solution can be made from 50 ml of 10N?

52. A solution contains 6 gm equivalents per liter of solution. What is its normality?

53. How much 3N HCl and 6N HCl must be mixed together to make 2 liters of 5N solution?

54. A procedure calls for 100 ml of 0.4N NaOH. 10N is on hand. How would one make 100 ml of 0.4N from what is on hand?

55. A $Hg(NO_3)_2$ solution to use in a titration chloride procedure is desired. What normality would one have to make so that each milliliter of the solution would be equal to 1 mg of chloride?

56. In a chloride procedure, 1 ml of $Hg(NO_3)_2$ solution equals 0.05 mg chloride. What is the normality of the titrating solution?

57. How many grams of HNO_3 will be contained in 100 ml of a 5N solution?

Specific gravity

Use the specific gravities and assays listed here for the following problems:

	sp gr	*%purity (assay)*
HCl	1.19	38
H_2SO_4	1.84	97
HNO_3	1.42	70

58. How many grams of HCl are in 100 ml of concentrated acid?
59. How many milliliters of H_2SO_4 would be required to make 400 ml of a 4M solution?
60. Given 30 ml of H_2SO_4 diluted up to 500 ml, what would be the percentage v/v and w/v?
61. How would one make 1000 ml of 6N HNO_3?
62. If there were 50 ml of HCl diluted up to 400 ml, give the following:
    a. $\%^{v/v}$
    b. $\%^{w/v}$
    c. Molarity
    d. Normality
63. Give the normality and molarity of the following:
    a. Concentrated HCl
    b. Concentrated H_2SO_4
    c. Concentrated HNO_3
64. A $10\%^{v/v}$ solution of HCl is available. How much concentrated HCl must be added to 500 ml of this 10% solution to make 1000 ml of 5N HCl?
65. $30\%^{w/v}$ H_2SO_4 is equal to what $\%^{v/v}$?
66. To make 130 ml of $10\%^{v/v}$ HCl from $20\%^{w/v}$, how much water would be needed?

Concentration relationships

67. Express 500 mg/dl NaCl as mEq/l Cl.
68. Express 90 mEq/l Na as mg/dl NaCl.
69. How much 6N HCl could be made from 20 ml of 12M HCl?
70. How much 3M H_2SO_4 can be made from 10 ml of 6N H_2SO_4?
71. 60 ml of 0.2N H_2SO_4 will make how much $20\%^{w/v}$ H_2SO_4?
72. 3N HCl is equal to what $\%^{w/v}$ HCl?
73. 20% HNO_3 is equal to what normal HNO_3 and what molar?
74. Express the following as mEq/l:
    a. 10 mg/dl Ca
    b. 700 mg/dl NaCl
    c. 14 mg/dl K
75. 0.85% saline is equal to what normality?
76. Express the following as mg/dl:
    a. 140 mEq/l Na
    b. 5 mEq/l Ca
    c. 5 mEq/l K
77. 20 ml of 6N H_2SO_4 will react with how many milliliters of 10% NaOH?
78. 100 ml of 3N NaOH will neutralize how many milliliters of $10\%^{v/v}$ HCl?
79. 30% NaOH is equal to what normality?
80. 1.7M HNO_3 is equal to what percentage?
81. How much 5M NaOH can be prepared from 50 ml of 10N NaOH?
82. 5N H_2SO_4 is equal to what molarity?
83. 3M H_3PO_4 is equal to what normality?
84. What is the concentration of 250 ml of 0.85% NaCl in terms of molarity and normality?

CHAPTER 7

Ionic concentration and pH

Many chemical reactions result from an interaction of charged particles. The charged particles are either atoms or molecules in which the total number of protons does not equal the number of electrons. Such particles of matter are called *ions*. Ions having more protons than electrons have a positive charge and are called *cations*. Ions having more electrons than protons have a negative charge and are called *anions*. Cations are attracted to anions by the electromagnetic forces associated with atoms and molecules. The attraction of two oppositely charge ions forms bonds between the particles. Such bond are called *ionic bonds*. A molecule formed from ions is stable if the positive charges equal the negative charges. When such compounds are not in solution, the molecules remain intact. Frequently, many of these molecules form interconnecting bonds to form crystals, which may be quite large.

When ionically bonded molecules are dissolved in a solvent having ionic bonds, the ions separate. Such separation is called *dissociation* or *ionization*. The most common solvent in which ions dissociate is water. Water itself ionizes to some degree. Two kinds of ions are formed from the ionization of water: hydrogen cations, H^+, and hydroxyl anions, OH^-. In a water solution, ions move away from one another, so that each ion can act independently. The only way in which most ions can undergo chemical reaction is to be dissociated.

In a particular water solution, different compounds dissociate to varying extents. The extent of dissociation of the substance determines what reactions will occur and the speed of those reactions. The rates of dissociation are influenced by the total complement of the ionic substances in the solution.

Three general types of ionic compounds exist: acids, bases, and salts. The complete description of each of these is beyond the scope of this book, but, stated simply and incompletely, acids are compounds that contribute hydrogen ions to a solution, bases are compounds that contribute hydroxyl ions to the solution, and salts are ionic compounds that yield neither hydrogen nor hydroxyl ions to the solution. An acid solution has more dissociated or free hydrogen ions than hydroxyl ions. A basic or alkaline solution has more free hydroxyl ions than free hydrogen ions. Those solutions in which the number of free hydroxyl ions is equal to the number of free hydrogen ions are said to be neutral solutions. All aqueous (water) solutions contain H^+ and OH^- ions. The degree of acidity or basicity of a particular solution depends on the relative concentration of the hydrogen and hydroxyl ions. Other ions affect this only indirectly. The acidity or basicity has a profound effect on the chemical reactions that occur in a solution. This effect involves the kinds of reactions and the speed of the reactions. Because of this, it is important to know the relative concentrations of the hydrogen and hydroxyl ions in a solution. One property of aqueous solutions is a great help in determining the concentration of ions. In all aqueous solutions, whether they are acid, basic, or neutral, the molar concentration of the hydrogen ions (designated $[H^+]$) multiplied by the molar concentration of the hydroxyl ions ($[OH^-]$) is always 1×10^{-14}. This fact shows that the concentration of hydrogen ions in a solution indicates the concentration of hydroxyl ions in the solution and vice versa. Hence, to indicate the degree of acidity or basicity of a solution one needs only to determine the concentration of either the dissociated hydrogen or hydroxyl ions. It is not necessary to determine both. In discussions of the degree of ionization of a solution, the concentration of the hydrogen ions is used for the measure. The probable reason for this is that 1 mole of hydrogen ion equals 1 gm. Hence, the molar concentration of a hydrogen ion solution is equal to the grams per liter of hydrogen.

$$[H^+] \times [OH^-] = 1 \times 10^{-14}$$

The H^+ concentration depends on the degree of dissociation or ionization; therefore, the degree of dissociation into ions will determine the relative strength of an acid or basic solution. The following formula may be used to determine the hydrogen ion concentration (in gm/l or M) when the normality and percent ionization (expressed as a decimal) are known.

$$N \times \% \text{ ionization} = [H^+]$$

Hydrogen chlorine is called a strong acid, for it will dissociate completely into H^+ and Cl^- in a dilute solution. The preceding formula could be used to find the H^+ concentration of a 0.1N HCl solution.

$$N \times \% \text{ ionization} = [H^+]$$
$$0.1 \times 1.0 \ (100\%) = 0.1 \text{ gm } H^+/l$$

Acetic acid is called a weak acid, for it will dissociate only slightly, about 1%, into hydrogen and acetate (CH_3COO^-) ions. For a 0.1N solution the H^+ concentration would be

$$N \times \% \text{ ionization} = [H^+]$$
$$0.1 \times 0.01 \ (1\%) = 0.001 \text{ gm } H^+/l$$

Trying to express the acidity or alkalinity of an aqueous solution by its H^+ concentration is quite often cumbersome and inconvenient.

Sørensen developed a scale to use in measuring this. He also created the symbol "pH" (which can be taken to mean *potence in hydrogen ion* or *potential of hydrogen ion*). He defined pH as the logarithm of the reciprocal of the H^+ concentration. Stated another way, pH is the negative logarithm of the molar concentration of the hydrogen ions.

Sørensen's scale permits the representation of the enormous range of the possible hydrogen ion concentration from a 1N (or M) H^+ to a 0.00000000000001N (or M) H^+ with numbers extending from 0 to 14.

Consider the scale presented in Table 5 and shown graphically in Fig. 7-1.

Notice in the acid column that as the H^+ decreases, the pH increases. Also, notice that each increase of one unit on the pH scale corresponds to a tenfold decrease in the H^+. Therefore, a change of $1/10$ or ten times in hydrogen ion concentration will make a change of 1 pH unit either up or down. The same holds true for bases. A change of either $1/10$ or ten times the base concentration will change the pH by 1 pH unit either up or down.

Recall that it was stated earlier that in all aqueous solutions the $[H^+] \times [OH^-]$ $= 1 \times 10^{-14}$.

	[H⁺]	**[OH⁻]**	
For a pH of 4.0	0.0001	$\times$ 0.0000000001	$= 10^{-14} = 1 \times 10^{-14}$
For a pH of 9.0	0.000000001	$\times$ 0.00001	$= 10^{-14} = 1 \times 10^{-14}$

From the preceding definition of pH, two formulas for pH and, similarly, two formulas for pOH are derived (see p. 75).

Table 5

[H⁺]	pH	[OH⁻]	pH
1.0 molar	0	0.00000000000001 molar	0
0.1	1	0.0000000000001	1
0.01	2	0.000000000001	2
0.001	3	0.00000000001	3
0.0001	4	0.0000000001	4
0.00001	5	0.000000001	5
0.000001	6	0.00000001	6
0.0000001	7	0.0000001	7
0.00000001	8	0.000001	8
0.000000001	9	0.00001	9
0.0000000001	10	0.0001	10
0.00000000001	11	0.001	11
0.000000000001	12	0.01	12
0.0000000000001	13	0.1	13
0.00000000000001	14	1.0	14

$$\left[H^+ \right]$$

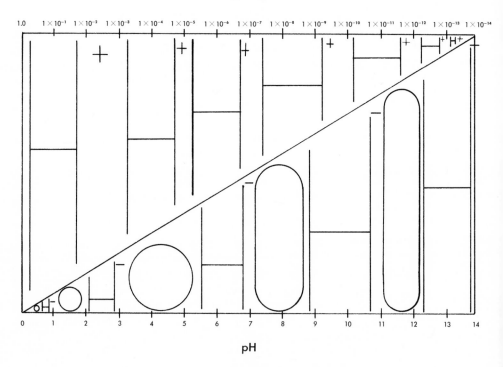

Fig. 7-1

pH	pOH

pH

1. $pH = \log \dfrac{1}{[H^+]}$

$pH = \log 1 - \log [H^+]$
$pH = 0 - \log [H^+]$
2. $pH = -\log [H^+]$

pOH

1. $pOH = \log \dfrac{1}{[OH^-]}$

$pOH = \log 1 - \log [OH^-]$
$pOH = 0 - \log [OH^-]$
2. $pOH = -\log [OH^-]$

In Table 6 notice again that the $[H^+] \times [OH^-] = 1 \times 10^{-14}$, but also notice that

$$pH + pOH = 14$$

This information may be used to solve certain types of problems. It is illustrated later in the chapter.

It can be shown that 10,000,000 l of water will yield 1 gm of H^+ or that 1 liter of water contains 1/10,000,000 gm of H^+. Since numbers such as these are large and unwieldy, they are often expressed as powers of 10.

$$10,000,000 = 10^7$$

$$\frac{1}{10,000,000} = \frac{1}{10^7} = 0.0000001 = 10^{-7}$$

For pure water the $[H^+]$ is 10^{-7}. Using the two preceding formulas for pH, it can be seen that the pH for pure water is as follows:

1. $pH = \log \dfrac{1}{[H^+]}$

$pH = \log \dfrac{1}{10^{-7}}$

$pH = \log 1 - \log 0.0000001$
$pH = 0 - \log 0.0000001$
$pH = -\log 0.0000001$
$pH = -(\overline{7}.0)$
$pH = -(-7.0)$
$pH = 7.0$

2. $pH = -\log [H^+]$

$pH = -\log 10^{-7}$

$pH = -\log 0.0000001$
$pH = -(\overline{7}.0)$
$pH = -(-7.0)$
$pH = 7.0$

Table 6

$[H^+]$	pH	pOH	$[OH^-]$
1.0 molar	0	14	0.00000000000001 molar
0.1	1	13	0.0000000000001
0.01	2	12	0.000000000001
0.001	3	11	0.00000000001
0.0001	4	10	0.0000000001
0.00001	5	9	0.000000001
0.000001	6	8	0.00000001
0.0000001	7	7	0.0000001
0.00000001	8	6	0.000001
0.000000001	9	5	0.00001
0.0000000001	10	4	0.0001
0.00000000001	11	3	0.001
0.000000000001	12	2	0.01
0.0000000000001	13	1	0.1
0.00000000000001	14	0	1.0

The relationship of pH to the hydrogen ion concentration can be expressed simply so long and the $[H^+]$ is equal to some negative power of 10. Such a value written in scientific notation would be 1×10^{-n}, where n equals some whole number between 1 and 14. The pH value for such a $[H^+]$ will equal the value of n, which is a whole number. The same relationship applies between the concentration of hydroxyl ions and pOH values. Pure water has a $[H^+]$ of 10^{-7}. This is equal to 1×10^{-7} or pH 7. In an earlier example, 0.1N HCl had a $[H^+]$ of 0.1 gm/l or 10^{-1} or pH 1. The 0.1N acetic acid had a $[H^+]$ of 0.001, 10^{-3}, 1×10^{-3}, or pH 3.

However, many solutions have a $[H^+]$ between exact negative powers of 10. The pH and pOH values of these must be calculated using logarithms. To calculate the pH or pOH value from the $[H^+]$ or $[OH^-]$, write the concentration using scientific notation. Then use the formula $a \times 10^{-b}$, when a equals the digits of the value and having a decimal point set between the first and second digit from the left and $-b$ equals the number of decimal places of the value. Study scientific notation in Chapter 1 if this is not clear.

EXAMPLE: $[H^+]$ expressed as $a \times 10^{-b}$

$$0.004 \quad = \quad 4.0 \times 10^{-3}$$

Substitute $a \times 10^{-b}$ in the formula for pH.

$$pH = -\log [H^+]$$
$$pH = -\log (a \times 10^{-b})$$
$$pH = -(\log a + \log 10^{-b})$$
$$pH = -(\log a + \bar{b})$$
$$pH = -[\log a + (-b)]$$
$$pH = -(\log a - b)$$
$$pH = -\log a + b$$
$$pH = b - \log a$$

This is another formula for pH that is important for calculations.

EXAMPLE: $[H^+] = 0.004$ gm/l; what is the pH of the solution?

$$[H^+] = a \times 10^{-b}$$
$$0.004 = 4 \times 10^{-3}$$

$$pH = -\log (a \times 10^{-b})$$
$$pH = -(\log 4 \times \log 10^{-3})$$
$$pH = -(\log 4 + \log 10^{-3})$$
$$pH = -(\log 4 + \log 0.001)$$
$$pH = -(\log 4 + \bar{3}.0)$$
$$pH = -[\log 4 + (-3.0)]$$
$$pH = -(\log 4 - 3.0)$$
$$pH = -\log 4 + 3.0$$
$$pH = 3.0 - \log 4$$
$$(b - \log a)$$
$$pH = 3.0 - 0.6021$$
$$pH = 2.3979$$

IN REVIEW: At this point, review the formulas presented thus far for pH (and similarly for pOH). The formulas indicated by the asterisks are the most common.

pH	**pOH**
*pH $= \log \dfrac{1}{[H^+]}$	*pOH $= \log \dfrac{1}{[OH^-]}$
pH $= \log 1 - \log [H^+]$	pOH $= \log 1 - \log [OH^-]$
pH $= 0 - \log [H^+]$	pOH $= 0 - \log [OH^-]$
*pH $= -\log [H^+]$	*pOH $= -\log [OH^-]$

$$pH = -\log (a \times 10^{-b})$$
$$pH = -(\log a + \log 10^{-b})$$
$$pH = -[\log a + (-b)]$$
$$pH = -(\log a - b)$$
$$pH = -\log a + b$$
$$*pH = b - \log a$$

$$pOH = -\log (a \times 10^{-b})$$
$$pOH = -(\log a + \log 10^{-b})$$
$$pOH = -[\log a + (-b)]$$
$$pOH = -(\log a - b)$$
$$pOH = -\log a + b$$
$$*pOH = b - \log a$$

Recall these known relationships for any ionic aqueous solution.

1. $[H^+] \times [OH^-] = 1 \times 10^{-14}$
2. $pH + pOH = 14$

EXAMPLE: A 0.1N acid solution is 70% ionized. Calculate the H^+ concentration.

$$N \times \% \text{ ionization} = [H^+]$$
$$0.1 \times 0.7 = 0.07 \text{ gm } H^+/l$$

EXAMPLE: What would be the pH of the preceding solution?

$$[H^+] = 0.07 \text{ gm/l}$$
$$0.07 = 7.0 \times 10^{-2}$$

$$pH = b - \log a$$
$$pH = 2 - \log 7.0$$
$$pH = 2 - 0.8451$$
$$pH = 1.1549$$

EXAMPLE: What would be the pOH of the solution in the two preceding examples?

$$pH + pOH = 14$$
$$1.1549 + pOH = 14$$
$$pOH = 14 - 1.1549$$
$$pOH = 12.8451$$

EXAMPLE: What would be the $[OH^-]$ in the preceding example?

$$[H^+] \times [OH^-] = 1 \times 10^{-14}$$
$$(7.0 \times 10^{-2}) [OH^-] = 1 \times 10^{-14}$$

$$[OH^-] = \frac{1 \times 10^{-14}}{7 \times 10^{-2}}$$

$$[OH^-] = \frac{1}{7} \times 10^{-12}$$

$$[OH^-] = 0.1428 \times 10^{-12}$$

EXAMPLE: An acid solution has 1/100,000 gm of H^+ per liter. Express this as pH.

$$\frac{1}{100,000} = 0.00001 = 10^{-5}$$

$$pH = -\log [H^+]$$
$$pH = -\log 10^{-5}$$
$$pH = -(\log 0.00001)$$
$$pH = -(\overline{5}.0)$$
$$pH = -(-5.0)$$
$$pH = 5.0$$

EXAMPLE: What is the $[H^+]$ of a solution having a pH of 8.95? Remember:

$$pH = \log \frac{1}{[H^+]} = b - \log a$$

In working problems of this type, the relationship between a and b is such that b may be any value and the $[H^+]$ will always be the same. The easiest way to work these problems is to assign *b* the value that is the smallest whole number that is equal to or greater than the pH or pOH value. In this problem *b* would equal 9.

$$8.95 = 9 - \log a$$
$$\log a = 9 - 8.95$$
$$\log a = 0.05$$
$$a = 1.12$$

$$[H^+] = a \times 10^{-b}$$
$$[H^+] = 1.12 \times 10^{-9}$$

The hydrogen ion concentration having a pH of 8.95 would be 1.12×10^{-9} moles/l.

If another value were used for *b* in the example, the result would be the same, as demonstrated in the following calculation:

$$pH = b - \log a$$
$$8.95 = 10 - \log a$$
$$\log a = 10 - 8.95$$
$$\log a = 1.05$$
$$a = 11.2$$

$$[H^+] = a \times 10^{-b}$$
$$[H^+] = 11.2 \times 10^{-10} = 1.12 \times 10^{-9}$$

EXAMPLE: To prepare 400 ml of a solution of NaOH with a pH of 12, how much NaOH would be needed?

NaOH is a strong base that dissociates completely.

$$NaOH \quad \rightarrow \quad Na^+ + OH^-$$

Since $[Na^+] = [OH^-] =$ the original [NaOH], in terms of molarity the molar concentration of OH^- will equal the molar concentration of the NaOH.

$$pH + pOH = 14$$
$$12 + pOH = 14$$
$$pOH = 14 - 12$$
$$pOH = 2$$

$$pOH = -\log [OH^-]$$
$$2 = -\log [OH^-]$$
$$2 = -\log (a \times 10^{-b})$$
$$2 = b - \log a$$
$$2 = 2 - \log a$$
$$\log a = 2 - 2$$
$$\log a = 0$$
$$a = 1.0$$

$$a \times 10^{-b} = 1.0 \times 10^{-2} = 0.01 \text{ moles/l NaOH}$$

$$0.01 \text{ moles/l} = 0.01\text{M solution}$$

$$\text{M} = \frac{\text{gm/l}}{\text{mol wt}}$$

$$0.01 = \frac{X}{40}$$

$$X = 40 \times 0.01$$
$$X = 0.4 \text{ gm/l}$$

It would take 0.4 gm to make 1 liter of this solution. However, the problem called for 400 ml; therefore: 0.4 gm is to 1000 ml as *X* gm is to 400 ml.

$$0.4 : 1000 = X : 400$$

$$\frac{0.4}{1000} = \frac{X}{400}$$

$$1000X = 160.0$$
$$X = 0.16 \text{ gm NaOH} \uparrow 400 \text{ ml} \rightarrow 400 \text{ ml of } 0.1\text{M Na OH}$$

EXAMPLE: Convert a $[H^+]$ of 0.45×10^{-9} to a pH value.

$$pH = b - \log a$$
$$pH = 9 - \log 0.45$$
$$pH = 9 - (\overline{1}.653)$$
$$pH = 9 - (-0.347)$$
$$pH = 9 + 0.347$$
$$pH = 9.347$$

In reality a logarithm consists of two numbers, the characteristic and the mantissa. Each of these numbers has its own sign: the characteristic being either negative or positive, whereas the mantissa is always positive. In the preceding example, log a consists of a negative characteristic and a positive mantissa. The pH value is expressed as a single number. To get a pH value, it is necessary to combine the values of the characteristic and the mantissa. If these two numbers carry the same sign (in which case they will both be positive), they are added, and there is no change in the logarithm.

EXAMPLE: Log $a = 1.216$.

$$
\begin{array}{rr}
\text{Characteristic} = & +1.0000 \\
\text{Mantissa} = & + \ .2160 \\
\hline
\text{Added together} & +1.2160
\end{array}
$$

If, however, the characteristic is negative, it is necessary to add the positive mantissa to the negative characteristic, and this produces one number with a negative sign.

EXAMPLE: Log $a = \overline{1}.653$.

$$
\begin{array}{rr}
\text{Characteristic} = & -1.0000 \\
\text{Mantissa} = & + \ .653 \\
\hline
\text{Added together} & - \ .347
\end{array}
$$

The negative characteristic and the positive mantissa were combined by algebraic addition to form the single negative number. Remember that such a number does not exist in a table of logarithms.

Frequently in calculations using logarithms, a single negative number results. The antilog of such a number cannot be found in this form. It becomes necessary to make a characteristic and a mantissa from the number. To do this, one may add a $+1$ then a -1 to the number.

EXAMPLE: Log $a = -0.95$.

This number cannot be found in a log table, because the mantissa *must* be positive. Add $+1$:

$$
\begin{array}{r}
1.000 \\
-0.95 \\
\hline
+0.05
\end{array}
$$

Add -1: $-1 + 0.05$. The -1 becomes the characteristic and the $+0.05$ becomes the mantissa ($\overline{1}.05$).

$$\log a = -0.95$$
$$\log a = \overline{1}.05$$
$$a = 0.112$$

ACID-BASE RELATIONSHIPS

The calculations involving the acid-base balance of the cells and fluids of the body involve some rather complex relationships that a book of this type should consider. The major buffer system of the body involves the following reactions:

$$CO_2 + H_2O \rightleftharpoons H_2CO_3 \rightleftharpoons H^+ + HCO_3^-$$

Carbon dioxide combines with water to form carbonic acid. Carbonic acid dissociates into hydrogen and bicarbonate ions. This system, in relation with the reactions of hemoglobin, maintains the pH of the body fluids at a remarkably constant value of 7.35 to 7.45.

All acids, bases, and salts ionize to a certain degree when dissolved in a solvent such as water. The proportion of the material that ionizes is called the *degree of dissociation*. When carbonic acid is dissolved in water, some of it ionizes into hydrogen and bicarbonate ions.

$$H_2CO_3 \rightleftharpoons H^+ + HCO_3^-$$

The law of mass action states that at a constant temperature the product of the concentration of the active substances on one side of a chemical equation when divided by the product of the concentration of the active substances on the other side of the chemical equation is a constant, regardless of the amounts of each substance present at the beginning of the reaction.

This means that the product of the hydrogen ion concentration times the bicarbonate ion concentration divided by the concentration of carbonic acid will always produce the same answer, no matter how much carbonic acid is added to a solution.

In other words, the degree of dissociation of a substance at a particular temperature will always be the same.

$$\frac{[H^+][HCO_3^-]}{[H_2CO_3]} = K'$$

It is extremely difficult to measure the concentration of carbonic acid directly. However, it has been found that in water solutions the molar concentration of dissolved carbon dioxide is 1000 times the molar concentration of carbonic acid.

$$[CO_2] = 1000 [H_2CO_3]$$

$$\frac{[H^+][HCO_3^-]}{[CO_2]} = K = \frac{1}{1000} K'$$

The CO_2 of this formula refers to the carbon dioxide dissolved in the blood plasma.

The hydrogen ion concentration can be calculated using a rearrangement of the preceding formula.

$$[H^+] = K \times \frac{[CO_2]}{[HCO_3^-]}$$

Because the hydrogen ion concentration is usually expressed as pH, it is usually more convenient to express all concentrations in this equation in the logarithmic form.

$$\log [H^+] = \log K + \log \frac{[CO_2]}{[HCO_3^-]}$$

Since pH $= -\log H^+$, change the signs of all logarithms.

$$-\log [H^+] = -\log K + \left(-\log \frac{[CO_2]}{[HCO_3^-]}\right)$$

Stated another way:

$$-\log [H^+] = -\log K + \log \frac{[HCO_3^-]}{[CO_2]}$$

Since $-\log H^+$ is called the pH, the $-\log K$ can be called the pK.

$$pH = pK + \log \frac{[HCO_3^-]}{[CO_2]}$$

This is one form of the Henderson-Hasselbalch equation. The pK value is constant only for a specific set of conditions. It varies inversely with the degree of dissociation, temperature, and pH. It varies with different solutions of the body. For example, the pK for serum and plasma is 6.10 at 37°C, whereas it is 6.18 for erythrocytes at this temperature.

Study of the Henderson-Hasselbalch relationship will show that an increase in the concentration of the bicarbonate ions will cause an increase in the pH of the solution. Similarly, an increase in the concentration of dissolved CO_2 will cause a decrease in the pH of the solution.

When a gas is dissolved in a liquid, the concentration of the gas in that liquid is directly proportional to the partial pressure of the gas. Hence, the dissolved carbon dioxide is proportional to the partial pressure of gaseous carbon dioxide. The partial pressure of CO_2 in mmoles Hg is designated by P_{CO_2}

$$[CO_2] = a \times P_{CO_2}$$

where a is the proportionality constant. This constant equals 0.0301 when the total carbon dioxide concentration is expressed as mmoles/l and 0.07 when the total carbon dioxide concentration is expressed ml%. If this information is added to the Henderson-Hasselbalch equation, the following formula results.

$$pH = pK + \log \frac{[HCO_3^-]}{a \times P_{CO_2}}$$

The total carbon dioxide is the dissolved CO_2 plus the bicarbonate ion. The small amount of carbonic acid is usually disregarded in these calculations.

$$\text{Total } CO_2 = [CO_2] + [HCO_3^-]$$

Remember, dissolved $CO_2 = a \times P_{CO_2}$. Hence:

$$\text{Total } CO_2 = a \times P_{CO_2} + [HCO_3^-]$$

If this formula is expressed differently:

$$[HCO_3^-] = \text{Total } CO_2 - a \times P_{CO_2}$$

Add this to the Henderson-Hasselbalch formula:

$$pH = pK + \log \frac{\text{Total } CO_2 - a \times P_{CO_2}}{a \times P_{CO_2}}$$

This form of the Henderson-Hasselbalch formula allows the calculation of any one of three values, pH, P_{CO_2}, or total CO_2. Recognize that two of the values must be known to calculate the third.

With the substitution of accepted values for pK (6.1) and a (0.03 for CO_2 in mmoles/l), the equation becomes

$$pH = 6.10 + \log \frac{\text{Total } CO_2 - 0.03 \text{ } P_{CO_2}}{0.03 \text{ } P_{CO_2}}$$

When the total CO_2 is expressed in millimoles per liter and the P_{CO_2} in mmoles Hg, the equation for expressing P_{CO_2} becomes

$$P_{CO_2} \text{ mmoles Hg} = \frac{\text{Total } CO_2 \text{ mmoles/l}}{0.03 \text{ [antilog } (pH - 6.1) + 1]}$$

The equation for determining the total CO_2 is

$$\text{Total } CO_2 \text{ mmoles/l} = 0.03 \text{ } P_{CO_2} \text{ [antilog } (pH - 6.1) + 1]$$

Using the preceding formulas and the following values, calculate each parameter.

$$pH = 7.44$$
$$P_{CO_2} = 37.7$$
$$CO_2 = 26$$

EXAMPLE: Determine the pH.

$$pH = 6.10 + \log \frac{\text{Total } CO_2 - 0.03 \text{ } P_{CO_2}}{0.03 \text{ } P_{CO_2}}$$

$$pH = 6.10 + \log \frac{26 - (0.03 \times 37.7)}{0.03 \times 37.7}$$

$$pH = 6.10 + \log \frac{26 - 1.131}{1.131}$$

$$pH = 6.10 + \log \frac{24.87}{1.131}$$

$$pH = 6.10 + \log 21.99$$
$$pH = 6.10 + 1.3422$$
$$pH = 7.44$$

EXAMPLE: Determine the P_{CO_2}.

$$P_{CO_2} = \frac{\text{Total } CO_2}{0.03 \text{ [antilog } (pH - 6.1) + 1]}$$

$$P_{CO_2} = \frac{26}{0.03 \text{ [antilog } (7.44 - 6.1) + 1]}$$

$$P_{CO_2} = \frac{26}{0.03 \text{ (antilog } 1.34 + 1)}$$

$$P_{CO_2} = \frac{26}{0.03 \text{ (}21.88 + 1)}$$

$$P_{CO_2} = \frac{26}{0.03 \times 22.88}$$

$$P_{CO_2} = \frac{26}{0.6864}$$

$$P_{CO_2} = 37.9$$

EXAMPLE: Determine the total CO_2.

$$\text{Total } CO_2 = 0.03 \text{ } P_{CO_2} \text{ [antilog } (pH - 6.1) + 1]$$
$$\text{Total } CO_2 = 0.03 \times 37.7 \text{ [antilog } (7.44 - 6.1) + 1]$$
$$\text{Total } CO_2 = 0.03 \times 37.7 \text{ (antilog } 1.34 + 1)$$

$$\text{Total } CO_2 = 0.03 \times 37.7 \, (21.88 + 1)$$
$$\text{Total } CO_2 = 0.03 \times 37.7 \times 22.88$$
$$\text{Total } CO_2 = 25.9$$

Another very common use of the Henderson-Hasselbalch equation is in the making of laboratory buffer solutions. The basic equation for this use is as follows:

$$pH = pK + \log \frac{[salt]}{[acid]}$$

In this formula the concentrations of the salt and the weak acid are usually expressed in moles per liter, millimoles per liter, or milliequivalents per liter. The pK values can be found in chemical reference books, such as the *Handbook of Chemistry and Physics*.*

EXAMPLE: Calculate the pH of an acetate buffer composed of 0.15M sodium acetate and 0.06M acetic acid. From a reference source the pK value for acetic acid is known to be 4.76.

$$pH = pK + \log \frac{[salt]}{[acid]}$$

$$pH = 4.76 + \log \frac{0.15}{0.06}$$

$$pH = 4.76 + \log 2.5$$
$$pH = 4.76 + 0.3979$$
$$pH = 5.1579$$
$$pH = 5.16$$

If the pK of the acid of a buffer pair and the total concentration of the buffer is known, the amount of salt and acid required to prepare a buffer can be calculated.

EXAMPLE: Prepare an acetate buffer whose concentration is 0.1M and buffers at a pH of 5.5.

The pK of acetic acid is 4.76, the molecular weight of acetic acid is 60, and the molecular weight of sodium acetate is 82.

$$pH = pK + \log \frac{[salt]}{[acid]}$$

$$5.5 = 4.76 + \log \frac{[salt]}{[acid]}$$

$$\log \frac{[salt]}{[acid]} = 5.5 - 4.76$$

$$\log \frac{[salt]}{[acid]} = 0.74$$

$$\frac{\text{moles/l salt}}{\text{moles/l acid}} = 5.5$$

These calculations show that the ratio of the moles per liter of salt divided by the moles per liter of acid is 5.5. Any ratio that gives this value may be used. One simple combination would be 5.5M salt and 1M acid. Remember that the ratio is based on molar concentration. This combination could be used only for buffer solutions having a total of 6.5 moles of buffer per liter of solution. However, the example calls for 0.1M. To find the amounts of buffer materials needed in a 0.1M buffer solution use the ratio-proportion procedure. The known ratio is 6.5 moles/l total buffer to 1 mole/l acetic acid. The desired system has 0.1 moles/l; hence

---

*Weast, R. C., editor: Handbook of chemistry and physics, ed. 54, Cleveland, Ohio, 1973, CRC Press.

$$\frac{6.5 \text{ total moles/l}}{1 \text{ mole/l acid}} = \frac{0.1 \text{ total mole desired}}{X \text{ acid}}$$

$$6.5X = 0.1$$
$$X = 0.015 \text{ moles/l acid}$$

Out of the total moles/l needed, 0.015 moles/l will be acid.

$$\text{moles/l acid} + \text{moles/l salt} = \text{Total moles/l}$$
$$\text{moles/l salt} = \text{Total moles/l} - \text{moles/l acid}$$
$$\text{moles/l salt} = 0.1 - 0.015$$
$$\text{moles/l salt} = 0.085 \text{ moles/l salt}$$

$$\text{moles/l acid} = 0.015\text{M}$$
$$\text{mol wt} \times \text{M} = \text{gm/l}$$
$$60 \times 0.015 = 0.9 \text{ gm/l}$$

$$\text{moles/l salt} = 0.9\text{M}$$
$$\text{mol wt} \times \text{M} = \text{gm/l}$$
$$82 \times 0.085 = 6.97 \text{ gm/l}$$

Therefore, 0.9 gm acid + 6.97 gm salt ↑ 1000 ml will yield 1 liter of 0.1M acetate buffer.

Practice problems

1. 10^{-9} equals which of the following:
   a. 0.00000009
   b. 0.000000001
   c. 0.000000009
   d. 0.0000001
2. A 0.6N acid solution is 80% ionized. Give the H^+ concentration.
3. A solution contains 1/100,000,000 gm H^+/l of solution. What is its pH?
4. If the $[H^+]$ is 1×10^{-6}, what is the $[OH^-]$?
5. Give the pH if the pOH is known to be 9.0.
6. A 0.03 acid solution is 70% ionized. Give each of the following:
   a. $[H^+]$
   b. $[OH^-]$
   c. pH
   d. pOH
7. How much HCl would be required to make 200 ml of a solution whose pH is 2.5.
8. Express the following as pH: $[H^+] = 3.1 \times 10^{-6}$.
9. Express the following as pH: $[H^+] = 0.54 \times 10^{-3}$.
10. Express the following as $[H^+]$: pH = 7.8.
11. Express the following as $[H^+]$: pH = 2.96.
12. How would one prepare an acetate buffer, pH 0.2M, having a pH of 6.0; pK acetic acid = 4.76.

CHAPTER 8

Dilutions

Laboratory procedures in which an amount of one substance is added to another to reduce the concentration of one of the substances are referred to as dilutions. These procedures have many uses in the laboratory. There are also many problems on the part of the laboratory personnel in manipulating these procedures.

One common problem with dilution procedures in the laboratory is the ambiguity and confusion in the exact meaning of the word *dilution*. The most common use of this word is so many parts of that material being diluted *in* the total number of parts of the final product. A much less common use of the word dilution is so many parts of the material being diluted *plus* so many parts of diluent. This second definition is rarely used, and when this meaning is intended, the procedure should be carefully and completely explained. Unless otherwise stated, this work will use the meaning of dilution in which the amount of material is diluted in the total amount of the final solution.

One thing should be stated now and borne in mind throughout the chapter: *A dilution is an expression of concentration, not volume. Stated another way, a dilution indicates the relative amount of the substances in a solution.*

Another variation in the terminology of this area is in the method used to denote the magnitude of the dilution. Some instructions read, make a 1 in 10 dilution; another states, make a 1 to ten dilution, and another might say, make a 1/10 dilution. No matter how such instructions are stated, they should all mean the same thing. The key word is *dilution*. When the word dilution is used, it should mean the number of parts of that being diluted in a total number of parts. In other words, *a dilution usually means the volume of concentrate in the total volume of final solution.*

In dilution statements, the smaller number is the number of parts of the substance that is being diluted; the larger number refers to the total number of parts in the final solution, unless explicitly stated otherwise. Consider the following statements:

1. Make a 1 to 10 dilution of serum in saline.
2. Make a 1 in 10 dilution of serum in saline.
3. Make a 1 to 10 dilution of serum with saline.
4. Make a 1/10 dilution of serum with saline.
5. Make a 1:10 dilution of serum using saline.
6. Make a dilution of 1 part serum and 9 parts saline.
7. Make a dilution of 1 part serum to 9 parts saline.

All of these statements mean the same thing. Other variations can be made in the preceding statements, and the meaning is still retained. In all the preceding statements, the directions can be followed by combining 1 ml of serum with 9 ml of saline to make 10 ml of the final solution, by adding 2 oz of serum to 18 oz of saline, or by placing 10 dr of serum in a measuring vessel and adding enough saline to make 100 dr of the final product. In all cases, there is 1 part original substance in 10 parts final solution.

$$\begin{array}{r} 1 \text{ part serum} \\ +9 \text{ parts saline} \\ \hline 10 \text{ parts final solution} \end{array}$$

A word of caution, when using the preceding procedure, be sure the instructions refer to dilutions. Some directions may ask for the same preparation as the preceding one but may use the word ratio instead of dilution. When a ratio is requested, the numbers have a significant difference in meaning. These numbers refer to the materials of the ratio. They may be written in several ways, such as 1:9, 1 ÷ 9, 1 to 9, and 1/9. No matter how the ratio is written, the order of the numbers must correspond to the order of the sub- stances to which the ratio refers. For example, a 1:9 serum to saline ratio equals a 9:1 saline to serum ratio. Both of these ratios would be the same as a 1:10 dilution of serum in saline. Similarly, a solution of serum and saline having a 1/10 ratio of serum to total volume would equal a 1 in 10 dilution of serum with saline.

EXAMPLE: Consider the following statement: Dilute 3 ml of serum with 25 ml of saline.

To complete this direction, one would add 25 ml of saline to 3 ml of serum. Hence, the total volume of the final solution would be 28 ml.

$$\begin{array}{r} 3 \text{ ml serum} \\ +25 \text{ ml saline} \\ \hline 28 \text{ ml final solution} \end{array}$$

The dilution of this solution would be 3 to 28. However, dilutions are usually stated as 1 to some number. To convert a 3:28 dilution to a 1 to something dilution, set up a ratio-proportion problem: 3 is to 28 as 1 is to X.

$$\frac{3}{28} = \frac{1}{X}$$
$$3X = 28$$
$$X = 9.33$$

3:28 dilution = 1:9.33 dilution

The serum to saline *ratio* in this example is 3:25 or 1:8.33, found as follows:

$$\frac{3}{25} = \frac{1}{X}$$
$$3X = 25$$
$$X = 8.33$$

3:25 ratio = 1:8.33 ratio

Another way to state this ratio is as a 25 to 3 saline to serum or 8.33 to 1 saline to serum ratio.

EXAMPLE: 5 ml of serum is diluted to 25 ml with saline. What is the serum dilution? What is the serum to saline ratio?

Set up the problem as 5 ml serum + X ml saline = 25 ml of the final solution.

$$X = 25 - 5$$
$$X = 20 \text{ ml saline}$$

The serum dilution is the amount of serum in the amount of total solution; hence, this is a 5:25 serum dilution. Reduce this to a 1 to X dilution.

$$\frac{5}{25} = \frac{1}{X}$$
$$5X = 25$$
$$X = 5$$

Hence, a 5:25 dilution would equal a 1:5 dilution. The serum to saline ratio would equal 5:20 or 1:4.

The preceding examples are presented in this manner for purposes of explanation. This should not be taken to mean that a dilution is always made by adding a given amount of one substance to a given amount of another substance. Quite the contrary, a dilution is usually made by taking the specified amount of the solution or substance to be diluted and adding enough of the diluent to make the desired volume of the final solution. The main reason for this is that 1 part of one substance plus 1 part of another substance does not always equal 2 parts of total volume. For example, 1 liter of water plus 1 liter of alcohol does not yield 2 liters of solution. It yields less than 2 liters because of the positioning of the molecules. For this reason, the suggested technique of diluting *up to* a final volume, rather than adding a designated amount, should be followed when applicable.

DILUTIONS AS AN EXPRESSION OF CONCENTRATION

Dilution notation is frequently used to express the concentration of solutions. Usually this method of expressing notation is used in connection with the titer of test solutions. Strictly speaking, *titer* is the concentration of a solution as determined by titration. Hence, the titer is the smallest amount or concentration that will produce a particular effect or endpoint.

EXAMPLE: A series of solutions of serum in saline is prepared in the following dilutions: 1:2, 1:4, 1:8, and 1:16. A test for the presence of an antibody was made on each solution. It was positive for the 1:2 and 1:4 dilutions but negative for the 1:8 and 1:16 dilutions. The titer of the antibody is said to be 1:4.

CALCULATIONS INVOLVING ONE DILUTION

The most common difficulties encountered in dilution procedures involve the calculations associated with the work.

EXAMPLE: Make 250 ml of a 1 to 10 dilution of serum in saline.

The final mixture in this problem has a *relative* concentration of 1 part serum in 10 parts of solution. The final volume of this solution would be 250 ml. Since an amount of serum is to be diluted up to a final volume with saline the amount of saline added need not be known. The simplest method to use in calculating the amount of serum is the ratio-proportion procedure.

$$\frac{1 \text{ part serum}}{10 \text{ parts solution}} = \frac{X \text{ ml serum}}{250 \text{ ml total solution}}$$

$$10X = 250$$
$$X = 25 \text{ ml}$$

Hence, to produce 250 ml of a 1 to 10 dilution of serum in saline, place 25 ml of serum in a measuring vessel and add enough saline to bring the total volume up to 250 ml.

EXAMPLE: Determine the amount of serum in 40 ml of a 1:5 dilution of serum in saline.

There is 1 part serum in every 5 parts of a 1:5 dilution.

$$\frac{1}{5} = \frac{X}{40}$$

$$5X = 40$$
$$X = 8$$

There are 8 ml of serum in 40 ml of a 1:5 dilution of serum with saline.

EXAMPLE: How much of a 1:16 dilution of urine in distilled water could be made with 3 ml of urine?

Again, using the ratio-proportion procedure

$$\frac{1 \text{ part urine}}{16 \text{ parts total volume}} = \frac{3 \text{ ml urine}}{X \text{ ml total solution}}$$

$$X = 16 \times 3$$
$$X = 48 \text{ ml}$$

Three milliliters of urine will make 48 ml of a 1:16 dilution of urine in distilled water.

Almost all other problems involving single dilutions can be solved by the proper use of the ratio-proportion procedure discussed in Chapter 1.

CALCULATIONS INVOLVING SEVERAL RELATED SOLUTIONS

Many laboratory procedures involve the use of a series of dilutions. A dilution series is a number of solutions made by diluting some substance with a solvent, then making a dilution of the resulting solution, and diluting this second solution to make a third, and so on. Extreme care must be taken in receiving or giving instructions pertaining to a dilution series. Occasionally dilution series may be described in which each dilution value refers to an independent dilution of some material in some solvent. More commonly, each value of a dilution series refers to a dilution of the previous solution. The meaning must be contained or clearly implied in the instructions concerning that particular dilution series.

EXAMPLE: Make the following dilutions of serum in saline: 1/5, 1/10, and 1/100.

In this example each of the three dilutions of serum is a separate and independent solution. To follow these instructions, one would make a 1/5 dilution of serum in saline, then a 1/10 dilution of serum in saline, and finally a 1/100 dilution of serum in saline.

EXAMPLE: A serum sample is diluted 1/5, rediluted 1/10, and again 1/100.

In this example each succeeding dilution is dependent on the previous solution in the series. A 1/5 dilution of serum is made with saline. This solution is diluted 1/10 with saline. The second solution is then diluted 1/100 with saline. Each is dependent on the previous operation.

The worker should be able to calculate the value of several properties of each step in a dilution series. Some of these values are as follows:
1. *Concentration* of material in each solution
2. Actual *amount* of material in each solution
3. Total *volume* of each solution

THE CONCENTRATION OF MATERIAL IN EACH SOLUTION

There are two areas of consideration to be used in dilutions, either in series or singly. One is how each dilution is made; the other is what each dilution contains. The important consideration is the concentration of the materials in the dilution. However, it is usually necessary to know how a dilution was made to figure the concentration of the materials in the dilution.

A general rule to use in calculating the concentration of solutions in a series is to multiply the original concentration by the first dilution, this by the second dilution, this by the third dilution, and so on until the final concentration is known.

EXAMPLE: A 5M solution of HCl is diluted 1/5. The resulting solution is diluted 1/10. Determine the concentration of each of the three solutions.

In this example, one solution is made from a solution that was made from another. To calculate the concentration of any of the solutions in such a series, express all dilutions as a fraction. Then multiply the concentration of the beginning solution by the dilution used in each succeeding step. The following steps are used in solving this example:

Step 1. The concentration of the first solution is given as 5M HCl. This then is the first answer.

Step 2. The second solution was made by a 1/5 dilution of the first solution. The concentration of HCl in the second solution would be calculated by multiplying the concentration of the first solution by the dilution used to produce the second solution.

$$5\text{M HCl} \times \frac{1}{5} = \frac{5}{5}\text{M} = 1\text{M}$$

Hence, the second solution has an HCl concentration of 1M.

Step 3. To calculate the concentration of HCl in the third solution in the series multiply the original concentration of HCl by the value of each succeeding dilution.

$$X = \text{conc of HCl in the last solution}$$

$$X = 5\text{M} \times \frac{1}{5} \times \frac{1}{10}$$

$$X = \frac{5}{50}$$

$$X = \frac{1}{10}\text{M}$$

The concentration of HCl in the last solution is 0.1M.

Notice that in each solution of this problem the concentration is expressed in molarity. This is because the concentration of the original solution was measured in molarity. In this type problem the concentration of each dilution will be expressed in the same form as that used in the original solution.

EXAMPLE: A 1/10 *dilution* of a substance is diluted 3/5, rediluted 2/15, and diluted once again 1/2. What is the final concentration?

$$\frac{1}{10} \times \frac{\overset{1}{\cancel{3}}}{5} \times \frac{2}{\underset{5}{\cancel{15}}} \times \frac{1}{\cancel{2}} = \frac{1}{250} \text{ dilution}$$

EXAMPLE: A 3% solution is diluted 2/30. What is the resulting concentration?

$$\cancel{3} \times \frac{2}{\underset{\underset{5}{10}}{\cancel{30}}} = \frac{1}{5}\% \text{ (or 0.2\%)}$$

EXAMPLE: A 6N solution is diluted 1/5, 1/2, 5/15, and 1/3. What is the final concentration?

$$\overset{2}{\cancel{6}} \times \frac{1}{\cancel{5}} \times \frac{1}{\cancel{2}} \times \frac{5}{15} \times \frac{1}{\cancel{3}} = \frac{1}{15}\text{N} \text{ (or 0.067N)}$$

EXAMPLE: A solution that contains 80 mg/100 ml is diluted 1/10 and again 2/20. What is the final concentration?

$$\frac{\overset{4}{\cancel{80}} \text{ mg}}{\underset{25}{\cancel{100}} \text{ ml}} \times \frac{1}{\underset{5}{\cancel{10}}} \times \frac{2}{\cancel{20}} = \frac{1 \text{ mg}}{125 \text{ ml}} = 1 \text{ mg/125 ml}$$

Notice that the final answer is *always* in *exactly* the same form as the original substance or solution.

In some dilution series the original concentration seems to be missing. The usual reason for this is that the first dilution was made with an undiluted substance, such as concentrated HCl, dry NaCl, or absolute alcohol, or a pure complex solution such as serum or urine. In such cases the concentration value for the original material is 1, to denote the whole or pure state of the substance.

EXAMPLE: Serum is diluted 1/10 with saline, and this solution is rediluted 1/5. What is the concentration of serum in each solution?

The dilution of the original substance, serum, would be 1/1, in other words, a pure substance. Recall, to get the concentration of material in any solution of a dilution series, multiply the original concentration by the dilution of each succeeding solution, up to and including the one being considered. Hence, to calculate the dilution of serum in the first dilution, multiply the concentration or dilution of the original substance by the dilution of the first solution.

$$\frac{1}{1} \text{ dilution} \times \frac{1}{10} = \frac{1}{10} \text{ dilution of serum in saline}$$

To get the actual dilution of serum in the second solution, multiply the concentration of the original substance by the dilution of the first and second solutions.

$$\frac{1}{1} \text{ dilution} \times \frac{1}{10} \times \frac{1}{5} = \frac{1}{50} \text{ dilution (concentration of serum in second dilution)}$$

Note that it is not necessary to include the 1/1 in the calculations, as it does not have any effect on the result.

Again, be careful to understand what each concentration value means, whether it is a pure substance dissolved in some solvent or some prepared dilution that is being diluted further.

The calculation of the concentration of a solution in a series can be made from the closest previous solution in the series for which the concentration is known. It is not necessary to always begin with the first dilution in the series.

EXAMPLE: A urine sample is diluted 1/2 with distilled water, rediluted 1/4, 1/4, and again 1/4. What is the concentration of the third and fourth solutions?

One could find the concentration of the third solution in the following manner:

$$\frac{1}{2} \times \frac{1}{4} \times \frac{1}{4} = 1/32 \text{ dilution}$$

The concentration of the fourth solution could be obtained in one of two ways.
1. Beginning with the first dilution

$$\frac{1}{2} \times \frac{1}{4} \times \frac{1}{4} \times \frac{1}{4} = 1/128 \text{ dilution}$$

2. Using the concentration of the preceding solution, the third solution, whose concentration was 1/32 dilution

$$\frac{1}{32} \times \frac{1}{4} = 1/128 \text{ dilution}$$

MAKING A DILUTION SERIES

The calculations used to determine the concentration of each solution in a series may be used in reverse to produce a dilution series having prescribed concentrations at each step.

EXAMPLE: Make the following dilutions of serum in buffer: 1/10, 1/100, and 1/500.

In each of the preceding dilutions, the numerator, 1, refers to the number of parts of serum and the denominators, 10, 100, and 500, refer to the number of parts of the total solution. One way to satisfy the preceding instructions would be to make each dilution separately, always using pure serum and pure buffer. This will work if sufficient serum is available. However, often a serum sample is of limited volume, so that the use of one dilution to make another becomes expedient. To do this, complete the following procedure. Note the reason for each step and recognize the possibility of adjusting each step to meet some other situation.

1. To make the first dilution, that is, the dilution most concentrated in serum, place 1 part serum in a vessel and bring the total volume up to 10 total parts. This is a 1 to 10 dilution of serum in buffer. The parts can mean any multiple or fraction of any unit of measure so long as *parts* has the same meaning throughout the preparation of this *one* solution. For example, let 1 part equal 1 ml. This means that 1 ml of serum was brought up to 10 ml total volume with buffer. One could let 1 part equal 0.5 ml, 0.001 ml, 1 liter, and so on, as long as all related calculations are based on the same thing.

2. To make the 1/100 serum in buffer dilution using the first dilution, determine the dilution to be made of the 1/10 dilution of serum in buffer. Remember, the concentration of each step of a series equals the product of the concentration of each preceding step and the original concentration.

$$\frac{1}{100} = \frac{1}{10} \times \frac{1}{X}$$

$$\frac{1}{100} \times \frac{10}{1} = \frac{1}{X}$$

$$\frac{10}{100} = \frac{1}{X}$$

$$10X = 100$$

$$X = 10$$

In substituting 10 for X, one can see there is a 1/10 dilution. To 1 part of the first solution add enough buffer to bring this solution to 10 parts of total volume. The magnitude of the parts must be consistant within one solution. It is not necessary to use the same unit of measure as used in the preparation of the first solution. For example, 1 part equaled 1 ml in the first solution. In the second solution 1 part may equal 2 oz or any other multiple of any unit of measure.

3. To make the 1/500 dilution of serum in buffer, make a 1/5 dilution of the second solution using buffer.

$$\frac{1}{500} = \frac{1}{100} \times \frac{1}{X}$$

$$\frac{1}{500} \times \frac{100}{1} = \frac{1}{X}$$

$$\frac{1}{X} = \frac{100}{500}$$

$$\frac{1}{X} = \frac{1}{5} \text{ dilution}$$

In making the 1/500 dilution of serum in buffer, bring 1 part of the 1/100 dilution of serum in buffer up to 5 parts total volume.

Note that the concentration in each of the tubes retains the same form of description as the original solution. In this case the first solution was described in terms of a dilution, that is, a 1/10 dilution of serum in buffer.

This discussion has dealt with making a dilution series by considering one tube at a time. The concentration of each tube in a series can also be calculated by multiplying the dilution of a solution by the concentration of each tube. This can be done for each succeeding tube in the series. However, the concentration of each solution in a series may not be in question. Frequently only the concentration of the final solution need be known. In such cases the concentration of the last solution made can be calculated by multiplying the concentrations of the original substance by the dilution of each succeeding solution, including the final, or last solution. There is no need to calculate the concentration of each solution unless the worker wants to know it.

EXAMPLE: A 10% solution of NaCl in water was diluted 1:5. A 1:2 dilution was then made of the result of the first dilution. This solution was then diluted 1:10. What is the NaCl concentration of the last dilution?

$$X = \text{NaCl concentration of the third dilution}$$

$$X = 10\% \times \frac{1}{5} \times \frac{1}{2} \times \frac{1}{10}$$

$$X = \frac{10}{100}$$

$$X = \frac{1}{10}\% = 0.1\%$$

Hence, the concentration of NaCl in the final solution is 0.1%. The concentrations of the intermediate solutions are not known.

Determining the amount of material in a dilution series

Often one needs to know the actual amount of substance contained in some part of a dilution series. The volume of a solution within the series, the mass of some solute in one of the solutions, and the amount of solute transferred to another solution are all amounts that the laboratory worker may have to know to complete some procedure properly. In determining any amount within a dilution series, the worker must think carefully through the procedures used to produce the series. The number of possible ways to make a dilution series makes precise directions impossible in the methods of determining amounts within the series. However, some guidelines can be offered to aid these determinations.

Volume of each solution

The volume of the total solution is dependent on the method used in preparing the series.

The concentration needed for each solution in the series is established by the particular procedure. The amount of each solution prepared is influenced by the available glassware, laboratory space, the amount of some component of the series, and several other factors. Usually the amounts of any solution used in a laboratory procedure are less than 500 ml and often less than 1 ml. The amounts are frequently some irregular value. Because of these factors, the competent laboratory worker must think through the procedures carefully.

EXAMPLE: A 1/10 dilution of serum is diluted 1/10 and rediluted 1/100. What is the final volume of each dilution?

In completing this instruction, one must consider a practical volume of material in each solution. If 10 ml would be a convenient volume, one could place 1 ml of serum in a vessel and bring the total volume up to 10 ml. This would provide 10 ml of the first solution. To make the second solution, take 1 ml of the first solution and dilute this up to 10 ml. This gives 10 ml of a 1/10 dilution of the first solution. However, the total volume of the first solution is now 9 ml. This may not effect the test, but the worker should be aware of this. To make the third solution, which is described as a 1/100 dilution of the second solution, one would take 0.1 ml of the second solution and dilute it up to 10 ml. The 0.1 ml is arrived at in the following manner: A 1/100 dilution means there is 1 ml of that being diluted in a total volume of 100 ml. A total volume of 100 ml is not desired; only 10 ml is needed. Hence

$$\frac{1}{100} = \frac{X}{10}$$
$$100X = 10$$
$$X = 0.1$$

Therefore, 0.1 ml in a total volume of 10 ml is the same concentration as 1 ml in a total volume of 100 ml. Therefore, if 0.1 ml of the second solution is diluted up to 10 ml, the resulting solution would be a 1/100 dilution of the second solution. The volume of the second solution would now be 9.9 ml, as 0.1 ml was removed.

In determining the volume of any solution in a series, the worker needs only to determine what went into each solution and what came out. Common sense and simple arithmetic would then be used to calculate the volume.

Amount of solute

The actual amount of the dissolved substance in each solution of a dilution series can be calculated if the relative concentration and volume of the solution are known. Consider the preceding example. A 1/10 dilution of serum is diluted 1/10 and rediluted 1/100. The volumes of these three solutions are 9 ml, 9.9 ml, and 10 ml for the first, second, and third solutions, respectively. The concentrations of serum in the first, second, and third solutions are 1/10, 1/100, and 1/10,000, respectively. If it is not understood how these concentration values are established, review the first part of this chapter.

In calculating the *amount,* or volume, of serum in the first solution, remember that there is 1 part of serum for each 10 parts of total solution in a 1/10 dilution. There are 9 ml of this solution. Use a ratio-proportion procedure. If there was 1 ml in every 10 there would be X ml in 9.

$$\frac{1}{10} = \frac{X}{9}$$
$$10X = 9$$
$$X = 0.9$$

In the remaining 9 ml of the first solution, there are 0.9 ml of serum. To determine the amount of serum in the second solution, one could use the same procedure. Concentration = 1/100; volume present = 9.9 ml. If there was 1 ml serum in every 100 ml, then there would be X ml serum in 9.9 ml.

$$\frac{1}{100} = \frac{X}{9.9}$$
$$100X = 9.9$$
$$X = 0.099 \text{ ml}$$

The second solution contains 0.099 ml of serum.

The amount of serum in the third solution could be calculated in a similar manner. Concentration = 1/10,000; volume present = 10 ml. There is 1 ml serum in every 10,000 ml; therefore, there would be X ml serum in 10 ml.

$$\frac{1}{10,000} = \frac{X}{10}$$

$$10,000X = 10$$
$$X = 0.001 \text{ ml}$$

It is important in this type of calculation that the worker carefully think through what is being done. No set procedure will suffice in all situations.

SERIAL DILUTIONS

Many procedures call for a dilution series in which all dilutions after the first one are the same. This type of dilution series is referred to as a serial dilution. The methods and calculations discussed for any type of dilution series apply to serial dilutions. This procedure is used in producing a series of solutions having equal increments of variation.

EXAMPLE: A serum sample is diluted 1:2 with buffer. A series of five dilutions is made of this first dilution by diluting it 1:10, rediluting 1:10, and then three times more, each resulting solution then being a 1:10 dilution of the previous one in the series. The concentration of serum in each solution is as follows: 1:2, 1:20, 1:200, 1:2000, 1:20,000, and 1:200,000.

Dilution problems related to correction by using the reciprocal of the dilution

Occasionally a solution is too strong to be used as it is. For example, when one is performing manual blood counts, the blood contains too many cells to be counted without some dilution. When performing a given test, it may be found that the concentration of the substance being measured is too high for measurement without a dilution. In these cases the original substance or solution on which the test is being performed has been altered, and for this change a correction must be made.

The general rule for this type problem states: To correct for having used a dilution in a determination rather than the concentration called for, multiply the answer obtained times the reciprocal of the dilution made.

EXAMPLE: A blood sample is diluted 1/500; 300 cells are counted in the diluted sample. How many cells would there be in the blood before the dilution was made?

If a 1/500 dilution of blood was made, the diluted sample would contain only $1/500$ as many cells as the undiluted sample, or, stated another way, whole blood would contain 500 times the number of cells as the diluted specimen. Therefore, if the number of cells counted in the diluted sample is multiplied times 500 (dilution = $1/500$ and reciprocal = $500/1$ = 500), one would have the number of cells present in the undiluted specimen.

$$300 \times 500 = 150,000$$

EXAMPLE: A test on a urine sample is to be run. The concentration of the substance in the urine is too high to be determined with the present procedure. Make a 1:10 dilution of the urine sample and run the test on the diluted solution. The answer obtained is 50 mg/dl. What should be reported?

The 1:10 dilution of urine would contain one-tenth the amount of substance as undiluted sample, or the undiluted sample would contain ten times the quantity of substance as the diluted solution. Multiply the answer obtained times the reciprocal of the dilution made (dilution = $1/10$ and reciprocal = 10).

$$50 \times 10 = 500 \text{ mg/dl}$$

Dilution problems related to making large dilutions

The instructions indicate that a 1:10,000 dilution of a substance is to be made. This means 1 part of solute (substance being diluted) in a total volume of 10,000 parts. If a 1:10,000 dilution of serum in saline is being made, it could be done by taking 1 ml of serum and diluting it up to a total volume of 10,000 ml. However, it is rare that this quantity of a solution is needed. If the approximate volume needed is known, a dilution problem procedure may be used to determine how to make a smaller quantity or volume of the desired concentration. The preceding dilution of serum could be made in several ways:

1. Make a 1:10 dilution of serum, redilute 1:10, redilute 1:10, and redilute once more 1:10.

$$\frac{1}{10} \times \frac{1}{10} \times \frac{1}{10} \times \frac{1}{10} = \frac{1}{10,000} \text{ dilution}$$

This would produce 10 ml of a 1:10,000 dilution of serum in saline.

2. Make a 1:10 dilution of serum, redilute 1:10, and again 1:100.

$$\frac{1}{10} \times \frac{1}{10} \times \frac{1}{100} = \frac{1}{10,000} \text{ dilution}$$

This would yield 100 ml of a 1:10,000 dilution of serum in saline.

3. Make a 1:100 dilution of serum and redilute 1:100.

$$\frac{1}{100} \times \frac{1}{100} = \frac{1}{10,000} \text{ dilution}$$

This would give 100 ml of a 1:10,000 dilution of serum in saline.

Any combination of dilutions that will yield a final concentration of 1:10,000 may be used. The combination is determined in part by the glassware available and the volume needed.

To decide what dilutions to use, one needs to know several things:

1. Original concentration of the substance being diluted
2. Final volume desired
3. Final concentration desired
4. Number of dilutions to be made (at times)

EXAMPLE: A 1:200 stock solution of boric acid is on hand. The patient requires 50 oz of a 1:500 solution. How would the necessary amount be made, without making an excess?

Recall the general rule for determining the concentration of a dilution series.

Original conc × Dilution 1 × Dilution 2 × . . . = Final concentration

Fill in the known parts.

Original conc × Dilution 1 = Final conc (that desired)

$$\frac{1}{200} \times \text{(unknown)} = \frac{1}{500}$$

Recall that the volume of the last dilution in a dilution series is the volume of the final solution. It is known that 50 oz of the 1:500 solution are needed. Therefore, if 50 is inserted for the total volume of the dilution to be made, that will leave the amount to be diluted as the unknown or *X*.

$$\frac{1}{200} \times \frac{X \text{ oz}}{50 \text{ oz}} = \frac{1}{500}$$

$$\frac{X}{10,000} = \frac{1}{500}$$

$$500X = 10,000$$

$$X = 20$$

If 20 oz of the stock 1:200 solution were diluted up to 50 oz, 50 oz of the desired 1:500 solution would be present.

EXAMPLE: A stock standard whose concentration is 50 mg/dl is available, but 50 ml of a working standard whose concentration is 0.2 mg/ml is needed. How would one make the desired volume of solution with the needed concentration?

$$\frac{50 \text{ mg}}{100 \text{ ml}} \times \frac{X \text{ ml}}{50 \text{ ml}} = \frac{0.2 \text{ mg}}{1 \text{ ml}}$$

(Recall that the answer is in *exactly* the same form as the original substance.)

$$\frac{50X}{5000} = \frac{0.2}{1}$$

$$50X = 1000$$

$$X = 20$$

If 20 ml of the stock standard were diluted up to a total volume of 50 ml, there would result 50 ml of a working standard with a concentration of 0.2 mg/ml.

Practice problems

1. If 30 ml of saline is added to 2 ml of serum, what is the serum dilution? What is the serum to saline ratio?
2. Give the serum to saline ratio for the following dilutions:
   a. 1/10
   b. 3/27
   c. 6/9
   d. 40/50
3. Express the preceding dilutions in the proper manner.
4. Given a total protein of 7.5 gm%, an albumin of 3.5 gm%, and a globulin of 4 gm%, state the albumin/globulin (A/G) ratio three different ways.
5. Make a 1/10,000 dilution of serum in saline using three tubes or less, but never have more than 100 ml total volume in any one tube.

If one were asked to take 10N NaOH, dilute 1/10, redilute 1/5, and again 3/15 (problems 6 to 9):

6. Exactly what procedure should be followed?
7. What would be the volume of the final solution?
8. What would be the concentration of the final solution?
9. How much 10N NaOH would actually be present in the final solution?
10. A glucose standard contains 5 mg/ml. A 1/10 dilution of this standard would contain how much glucose per milliliter?
11. Given a series of ten tubes, each of which contains 5 ml diluent. To the first tube is added 1 ml serum, and a serial dilution using 1 ml is carried out in the remaining tubes. What is the serum concentration in tube 4 and 8?
12. A 20% solution is diluted 1:50. What is the volume and concentration of the final solution?
13. A 1/10 dilution is diluted 1/5 and again 1/5. What is the final dilution?
14. A 40:1000 stock solution of boric acid is available, and 50 oz of a 1:300 solution is needed. What procedure would be followed to make the desired volume and concentration?
15. 8 oz of a 1:500 solution of phenylephrine is needed for use with pediatric patients. A 1:100 solution used for adults is available. How would the needed solution be prepared?

CHAPTER 9

Colorimetry

The colorimeter is one of the most used analytical tools in the clinical laboratory. This instrument can be used in making qualitative and quantitative determinations of many biological materials. It works by measuring the kind and amount of light absorbed or transmitted by a substance. The materials tested in a clinical laboratory are usually in solution.

The wavelength determines the color of light. The color of a substance is determined by the wavelengths of the light transmitted from it. A colorimeter has a light source of known quality. The light is passed through a prism or a grating to separate the different wavelengths of light, resulting in individual color bands. Light of one wavelength is directed toward a vessel holding a solution of the material being examined. The amount of light allowed to pass through the solution is measured by a photometer as either the absorbance or the percent transmittance.

For a complete explanation of the mechanics and theory of operation of a colorimeter consult one of the standard texts listed at the end of the book.

There are several calculations involved in the use of colorimetry in the laboratory, particularly involving the use of curves and standards. The law forming the mathematical basis for colorimetry is really a combination of several laws often collectively called *Beer's law*. Stated simply it says that the absorbance, A, of a colored solution is equal to the product of the concentration of the color-producing substance, C, times the depth of the solution through which the light must travel, L, times a constant K. Written as an equation, this law becomes the following:

$$A = C \times L \times K$$

It is from this relationship that some of the formulas are derived. There are two main types of colorimetry: (1) visual and (2) photometric. Visual colorimetry is seldom used and will be presented here only as a mathematical contrast to photometric colorimetry.

VISUAL COLORIMETRY (INVERSE COLORIMETRY)

In visual colorimetry the colors of a standard solution and an unknown solution are set equal to each other by varying the depth of solution through which one looks. The color is an indication of the absorbance of the solutions. Referring to the mathematical equation of Beer's law, $A = C \times L \times K$, there will be one formula that refers to the standard and one that refers to the unknown.

Standard	Unknown
$A_s = C_s \times L_s \times K$	$A_u = C_u \times L_u \times K$

Since A_s has been set to equal A_u it can be said that $A_s = A_u$. If this is true, then, substituting for A_s and A_u, one would have the following:

$$A_s = A_u$$
$$C_s \times L_s \times K = C_u \times L_u \times K$$

97

Since K appears on both sides of the equation, it may be cancelled out.

$$C_s \times L_s = C_u \times L_u$$

The concentration of the unknown is to be determined; therefore, the following should be set up:

$$C_u \times L_u = C_s \times L_s$$

$$C_u = \frac{C_s \times L_s}{L_u}$$

$$C_u = \frac{L_s}{L_u} \times C_s$$

Visual colorimetry is referred to as *inverse* colorimetry because as the reading, L_u, of the unknown increases, the concentration of the unknown, C_u, decreases.

PHOTOMETRIC COLORIMETRY (DIRECT COLORIMETRY)

In photometric colorimetry the depth of the solution is held constant (cuvette diameter determines the depth), and the absorbance changes (the reading taken from the instrument). Here, again, there will be one formula for the standard and one for the unknown.

Standard	**Unknown**
$A_s = C_s \times L_s \times K$	$A_u = C_u \times L_u \times K$

In photometric colorimetry the depth is held constant, and the absorbances vary and are read from a scale; therefore

$$L_s = L_u$$

$$L_s = \frac{A_s}{C_s \times K} \qquad\qquad L_u = \frac{A_u}{C_u \times K}$$

therefore

$$\frac{A_s}{C_s \times K} = \frac{A_u}{C_u \times K}$$

or since K appears on both sides

$$\frac{A_s}{C_s} = \frac{A_u}{C_u}$$

$$\frac{C_u}{A_u} = \frac{C_s}{A_s}$$

$$C_u = \frac{C_s}{A_s} \times A_u$$

$$C_u = \frac{A_u}{A_s} \times C_s$$

Photometric colorimetry is called *direct* colorimetry because as the absorbance of the unknown, A_u, increases, the concentration of the unknown, C_u, also increases.

This formula applies *only* when Beer's law is followed. If it is followed, the absorbance and concentration will be directly related; that is, if the absorbance doubles, the concentration doubles; if the absorbance triples, the concentration triples; and so on. Some solutions do not show this relationship. In such cases, a standard curve must be used to determine the concentration of the unknown (see Chapter 10).

RELATIONSHIP BETWEEN ABSORBANCE AND %*T*

Look at the relationship between *A* (or *OD*, optical density) and %*T* presented in Fig. 9-1.

In Fig. 9-1 the divisions on the absorbance scale are unequal and almost impossible to separate on the left side. *Absorbance, A,* is a measure of the amount of light stopped, or absorbed, by a solution, and the absorbance of light is a logarithmic function; hence, the *A* scale is a logarithmic scale. On the other hand, *transmittance* (Fig. 9-2) is a measure of the amount of light allowed to pass through a solution. Since *transmission* is a mathematical comparison of the amount of light emerging from a solution to the amount of light entering the solution and since *transmittance value* is the comparison of the transmission of the unknown solution to the transmission of the blank solution, the %*T* scale is a linear scale. Since the divisions on the %*T* scale are equally spaced and easy to read, these divisions are commonly seen on most instruments. Because the following relationship is true, *A* = light stopped and *T* = light passed through, *A* and *T* are inversely related. Because the absorption of light is a logarithmic function, they are also logarithmically related. Therefore, the following is the basic relationship between *A* and *T*:

$$A = \log \frac{1}{T}$$

This relationship may be rearranged to give a second relationship.

$$A = \log \frac{1}{T} \text{ (first relationship)}$$

$$A = \log 1 - \log T$$
$$A = 0 - \log T$$
$$A = -\log T \text{ (second relationship)}$$

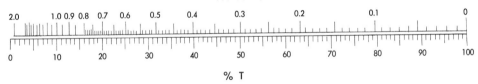

Fig. 9-1

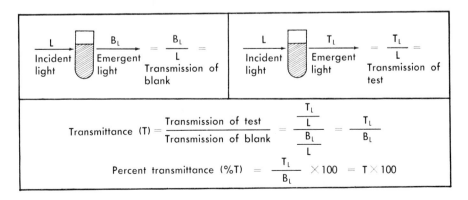

Fig. 9-2

With a little substitution, the most commonly seen relationship may be derived.

$$\%T = T \times 100$$

Therefore

$$T = \frac{\%T}{100}$$

If $\%T/100$ is substituted for T in the second relationship, the following become apparent:

$$A = -\log \frac{\%T}{100}$$

$$A = -(\log \%T - \log 100)$$
$$A = -(\log \%T - 2)$$
$$A = -\log \%T + 2$$
$$A = 2 - \log \%T \text{ (third relationship)}$$

Beginning with the first basic relationship, it is possible to derive the other two most commonly stated relationships (denoted by *) as follows:

$$*A = \log \frac{1}{T}$$

$$A = \log 1 - \log T$$
$$A = 0 - \log T$$
$$*A = -\log T$$

$$A = -\log \frac{\%T}{100}$$

$$A = -(\log \%T - \log 100)$$
$$A = -(\log \%T - 2)$$
$$A = -\log \%T + 2)$$
$$*A = 2 - \log \%T$$

In the course of everyday work, these relationships are the ones that laboratory workers will come in contact with most often. Learn them. Understand them. They will be used in the next chapter.

ABSORBANCE AND ITS RELATIONSHIP TO MOLAR ABSORPTIVITY

Colorimetry can be used to determine the actual concentration of materials in solution rather than simply a relative concentration. To do this the absorbance of a solution must be used in connection with a known coefficient for the particular compound being measured at a particular wavelength. This coefficient is known as the molar absorptivity (also knows as ϵ, molar absorption coefficient, and molar extinction coefficient) and is usually the absorbance (at a given wavelength) of a 1M solution of the pure substance through a 1-cm light path. Stated another way, the absorbance is the product of absorptivity, the optical light path, and the substance concentration (usually in moles/l). Molar absorbance coefficients for the substances being tested can usually be found from references. This coefficient can also be used to estimate the purity of the dissolved material.

To use the molar absorptivity for concentration determinations, one can include the results for a test in the following formula to calculate the concentration of the material in the sample:

$$A = \epsilon \times c \times d$$

where A is the absorbance of the sample at a given wavelength; ϵ, the molar absorptivity; c, the concentration in moles per liter; and d, the length of the light path in centimeters.

EXAMPLE: If ϵ is known, the concentration can be calculated from the absorbance.

$$c = \frac{A}{\epsilon \times d}$$

Since $d = 1.0$

$$c = \frac{A}{\epsilon}$$

The ϵ of nicotinamide adenine dinucleotide (NADH) for three different wavelengths is as follows: 340 nm = 6.22×10^3, 366 nm = 3.3×10^3, and 334 nm = 6.0×10^3. The absorbance values at these wavelengths were found to be 340 nm = 0.311, 366 nm = 0.165, and 334 nm = 0.300. Insert these values to calculate the concentration of the solution.

$$\text{(at 366 nm) } c = \frac{0.165}{3.3 \times 10^3} = 0.05 \times 10^{-3} \text{ moles/l}$$

$$\text{(at 340 nm) } c = \frac{0.311}{6.22 \times 10^3} = 0.05 \times 10^{-3} \text{ moles/l}$$

$$\text{(at 334 nm) } c = \frac{0.300}{6.0 \times 10^3} = 0.05 \times 10^{-3} \text{ moles/l}$$

One can determine the purity of a solution of known concentration by calculating the molar absorptivity if the concentration and absorbance values are known; this is then compared to the value for the pure substance. The following is a convenient formula for this determination:

$$\epsilon = \frac{A}{c \times d}$$

Since $d = 1.0$

$$\epsilon = \frac{A}{c}$$

EXAMPLE: A solution of NADH has a concentration of 0.05×10^{-3} moles per liter. What would the ϵ be at 340 nm, 366 nm, and 334 nm using the absorbance values from the preceding example?

Using these values, one obtains the following information:

$$\epsilon_{366} = \frac{0.165}{0.05 \times 10^{-3}} = 3.3 \times 10^3$$

$$\epsilon_{340} = \frac{0.311}{0.05 \times 10^{-3}} = 6.22 \times 10^3$$

$$\epsilon_{334} = \frac{0.300}{0.05 \times 10^{-3}} = 6.0 \times 10^3$$

One can further derive that the amount of NADH reduced in a reaction can be computed from the measured change in absorbance, ΔA.

EXAMPLE: Using the preceding values, if a change in absorbance of 1.000 is obtained at the three wavelengths, one would find that the concentration of NADH is the following:

$$\Delta A_{340} = 1.000$$

$$c = \frac{1.000}{6.22 \times 10^3} = 1.608 \times 10^{-4} \text{ moles/l}$$

$$\Delta A_{366} = 1.000$$

$$c = \frac{1.000}{3.3 \times 10^3} = 3.030 \times 10^{-4} \text{ moles/l}$$

$$\Delta A_{334} = 1.000$$

$$c = \frac{1.000}{6.0 \times 10^3} = 1.667 \times 10^{-4} \text{ moles/l}$$

Before these coefficients can be used with most analytical instruments, they must be adjusted to conform to the range of the instrument. This is done by diluting the sample and then making a mathematical correction of the results. For example, a 1M solution of bilirubin, suitable for use as a standard, should have an absorbance of 60,700 (mean) ± 800 at 453 nm in chloroform at 25°C, when measured in a cuvette with a 1 cm light path. Since the most accurate range in spectrophotometry is approximately 0.2 to 0.8 A, the dilution should be made so that readings will fall within these limits. If a 1M solution had an absorbance of 60,700 a 1/60,700M (a 1/60,700 dilution of a 1M) would have an absorbance of 1.0. Hence, a 1/121,400M solution would have an absorbance of 0.5, which is within the desired range.

If the instrument being used has a light path of other than 1 cm, correction must be made for this difference.

EXAMPLE: What would be the molar absorptivity of a 1M solution of bilirubin diluted 1:121,400 and giving an absorbance of 0.73 on a machine using a light path of 1.5 cm?

$$\epsilon = \frac{A}{c \times d}$$

$$\epsilon = \frac{0.73}{\dfrac{1}{121,400} \times 1.5}$$

$$\epsilon = 59,350 \text{ (which would not be within the acceptable range)}$$

Practice problems

Derive the following from Beer's law ($A = C \times L \times$ K):

1. The short formula for visual colorimetry
2. The short formula for photometric colorimetry

3. Give three (and derive two) relationships between A and %T.

Define the following:

4. Absorbance
5. Transmission
6. Transmittance value
7. %T

CHAPTER 10

Standard curves

Many procedures conducted in clinical and biological laboratories involve the use of standard curves. A standard curve as used in this connotation is a line plotted on graph paper; this line reflects the pattern of values from a test procedure or instrument in response to variations in the concentration of the material being tested. This curve is usually established by using several known values of the test material.

Once this curve is established, it is used in several ways: (1) It may be used to determine an unknown value. This is probably the most common use of standard curves in most laboratories, that is, the determination of concentration by colorimetric procedures. The general principle governing the pattern of variation of most procedures is Beer's law. Remember, Beer's law may be expressed as $A = C \times L \times K$. In other words, absorbance is directly proportional to concentration. If the cause of the variation of the absorbance values does not conform to Beer's law, the formula

$$C_u = \frac{A_u}{A_s} \times C_s$$

for the determination of the concentration of the unknown value may not be used and a standard curve must be made. (2) If many test determinations are performed at one time, it is an arduous task to calculate each one using the formula; hence, a standard curve may be used to expedite the completion of a large number of similar tests. (3) Still another common use of standard curves is to determine if a series of values conforms to some general principle. In this respect, a standard curve may be used to determine if a new or unknown procedure conforms to Beer's law.

The details of the formulation of a standard curve will vary with each procedure. However, there are some general guidelines to follow. (1) The range of values on the curve should correspond to the most efficient range of the test system or instrument. (2) The curve should be based on at least three known values. This is a minimum. More should be used where possible. For most procedures a good curve can be produced from five to seven well-distributed points. (3) If possible, the values of each end of the curve should be beyond the values of any unknown used with the curve. (4) As with most endeavors of life, common sense and sound logic must be used in the development and use of a standard curve.

Because the most common use of standard curves is to convert colorimeter readings to concentrations of materials in solution, the rest of the chapter will deal principally with the procedures relating to this use.

Colorimetric values reflect a color intensity of the solution placed in the light path of the machine. The color intensity is related to the amount of the color producing substance in the light path. If the distance of the path of light through the solution is constant, the *concentration* of the test solution is the property that determines the amount of material in the light path. In general, the same concentration of a given material will produce the same response by the machine. The meaning of any concentration measurement is determined by the procedures used to obtain the concentration.

The points on which a standard curve is drawn are based on the response of the colorimeter to the known concentrations of a series of standard solutions. To greatly increase the convenience of a curve, it is necessary that the concentration notation on the graph be in terms of the equivalent concentration of the material on which the tests are to be made. For example, if a standard curve is made for the determination of milligrams of glucose per deciliter of blood, then the concentration notation on the graph should be in terms of milligrams of glucose per deciliter of blood and not in the concentration of the standard solutions used to establish the curve.

The methods used to adjust the standard concentrations to concentrations of the test material depends on the procedures used in the preparation of the solution for use in the colorimeter. One of the most complex of such adjustments is that needed when simple aqueous solutions are used as the standard solution for the establishment of a standard curve to be used for serum concentration determinations. The following formula for this adjustment is given in some textbooks:

$$C_u = \frac{A_u}{A_s} \times \left[W_s \times \frac{V_u}{V_s} \times D \times \frac{V_c}{V_t} \right]$$

where C_u is the concentration of the test (unknown) solution; A_u, the absorbance of the test solution; A_s, the absorbance of the standard solution; W_s, the total weight (mass) of the standard substance used; V_u, final volume of the test solution; V_s, final volume of the standard solution; D, a factor to correct for any dilution made in the test sample, that is, serum, blood, or urine; V_c, volume base of the reported values; and V_t, volume of test solution taken for analysis.

On first examination this could be accurately termed an unholy mess. However, if careful study is made of each part of this formula some sense can be made of it. This formula is an expanded form of the one used for the practical expression and use of Beer's law.

$$C_u = \frac{A_u}{A_s} \times C_s$$

Note that the last portion of the long formula is simply an expression of the calculation of the concentration of the standard solution in terms compatible with a particular test procedure.

Remember that if the absorbance characteristics of the test substance do not conform to Beer's law, the formula cannot be used to calculate the concentration of an unknown solution. A standard curve has to be made. However, the points of the curve can be made equivalent to the concentration of the test material by using the latter part of the long formula.

$$C_s = W_s \times \frac{V_u}{V_s} \times D \times \frac{V_c}{V_t}$$

The W_s equals the total weight or the mass of the standard substance taken for color development. The mass of the standard substance used can be calculated by multiplying the number of milliliters of the working standard used by the amount of the substance per milliliter in the standard solution.

EXAMPLE: A working standard has a concentration of 10 mg/50 ml, and 2 ml of this working standard are used. What would the W_s be for this problem?

Concentration of working standard = 10 mg/50 ml = 1 mg/5 ml = 0.2 mg/ml. If 2 ml of this standard were used, there would be a total of

$$2 \times 0.2 \text{ mg} = 0.4 \text{ mg}$$
$$W_s = 0.4 \text{ mg}$$

The part of the formula designated D is the dilution factor, which corrects the calculation for any dilutions made of the test sample. See Chapter 8 for a discussion of dilution factors, if necessary, for a review of how to calculate a dilution factor.

The final volumes of the test and standard solutions (V_u and V_s, respectively) are the total volumes of the solutions at the end of the test procedure. Both of these volumes are usually the same. If this is the case, the result of this fraction (V_u/V_s) is one. This would have no effect on the final answer and can be deleted from the formula ($W_s \times D \times V_c/V_t$). If these two volumes are not equal, the result of the expression is something other than one and must be included in the calculation.

The factor V_c is equal to the volume on which the report of the test results is based. The concentration of substances in the body fluids is most often reported as parts per deciliter (100 ml) of fluid. For example, blood sugar concentrations are reported as milligrams of glucose per deciliter of blood or serum. In this kind of test, V_c would be equal to 100 (1 dl = 100 ml).

The part of the formula designated V_t is equal to the amount of the test sample used in the analysis. If a dilution has been made of the test sample, V_t refers to the volume of diluted sample used for color development and D is included in the formula to correct for the dilution that was made. If there has been no dilution of the test sample, V_t refers to the actual amount of test sample (such as, blood, serum, or urine) used and D would not be needed.

These three values (D, V_c, and V_t) correct the formula for differences in the reporting base (such as, milligrams per deciliter) and the volume of sample tested. If a test result for blood sugar is reported as 25 mg/dl, this means that there are 25 mg glucose/100 ml blood. However, 100 ml blood would not normally be taken for analysis. Usually, much less blood or sample is used. Hence, a correction is made for this difference by the inclusion in the formula of the following expression:

$$D \times \frac{V_c}{V_t}$$

A rearrangement of the last portion of the long formula ($W_s \times D \times V_c/V_t$) yields a simpler formula for everyday use in producing a standard of some desired concentration:

$$\text{ml std} \times \frac{100}{\text{Quantity of test sample}} \times \text{conc of } WS/\text{ml} = C_s$$

where ml std is the number of milliliters of the working standard used in the test procedure; 100 is used to produce results reported in percent concentration, such as mg/dl (if the results are to be reported in parts per liter, this factor is changed to 1000); quantity of test sample is the actual quantity (usually in milliliters) of the sample being tested before any alteration in volume (if procedures calling for filtrates or dilution are used, this is the actual amount of the test sample present in the final solution taken for analysis); conc of $WS/$ml is the concentration in parts per milliliter of the working standard; and C_s is the equivalent concentration of the standard with which one is working for *this* procedure.

NOTE: There is an important difference in the meaning of the terms *working standard* and *stock standard*. The stock standard, *SS*, refers to the solution that is normally stored, whereas the working standard, *WS*, is the solution used in the test procedure. These terms may refer to the same solution. However, on occasion, low concentrations of some materials are not stable; therefore, higher concentrations are used for storage. In these cases a dilution of the stock standard is made to produce a working standard with the desired concentration.

EXAMPLE: Making a working standard from a stock standard: the concentration of a stock standard is 1000 mg/dl; a working standard with a concentration of 0.2 mg/ml is desired.

$$SS = 1000 \text{ mg/dl}$$
$$SS = 1000 \text{ mg/100 ml}$$
$$SS = 10 \text{ mg/ml}$$

A dilution procedure may be used to figure out how to make the needed concentration. Set up the dilution problem by putting down the original concentration (what is on hand) and the final concentration (what is desired) and make the denominator of the first dilution the volume that is desired. If 100 ml of the preceding working standard is desired, the problem would be filled in as follows:

Available stock		Dilution needed		Desired concentration
$\dfrac{10 \text{ mg}}{1 \text{ ml}}$	$\times$	$\dfrac{X}{100}$	$=$	$\dfrac{0.2 \text{ mg}}{1 \text{ ml}}$

$$\frac{10}{1} \times \frac{X}{100} = \frac{0.2}{1}$$
$$10X = 0.2 \times 100$$
$$10X = 20$$
$$X = 2$$

A 2/100 dilution of the stock standard is needed, that is, 2 ml stock standard ↑ 100 ml would give 100 ml of a working standard with a concentration of 0.2 mg/ml. Another way to think about this type problem would be

$$SS = 1000 \text{ mg/dl}$$
$$SS = 1000 \text{ mg/100 ml}$$
$$SS = 10 \text{ mg/ml}$$

In every milliliter of stock standard there are 10 mg glucose. Set up a ratio and proportion as follows: 0.2 mg in 1 ml would be the same as 10 mg in X ml.

$$\frac{0.2 \text{ mg}}{1 \text{ ml}} = \frac{10 \text{ mg}}{X \text{ ml}}$$
$$0.2X = 10$$
$$X = 50$$

If there were 10 mg in 50 ml, the desired concentration would be attained. To get 10 mg in 50 ml take 1 ml stock standard (which contains 10 mg) and dilute this up to 50 ml. This would then be a concentration of 10 mg/50 ml or 0.2 mg/ml. Likewise, 2 ml stock standard diluted up to 100 ml = 20 mg/100 or 0.2 mg/ml. Use whichever method makes most sense to you!

Compare the two formulas:

$$W_s \times D \times \frac{V_c}{V_t} = C_s$$

$$\text{ml std} \times \frac{100}{\text{Quantity of test sample}} \times \text{conc WS/ml} = C_s$$

The W_s of the long formula is represented by the ml std and the conc of *WS*/ml because the product of the concentration per milliliter times the number of ml used is the total weight of standard used in the procedure.

$$D \times \frac{V_c}{V_t}$$

is represented by

$$\frac{100}{\text{Quantity of test sample}}$$

EXAMPLE: A 1:10 filtrate (dilution) is made in a serum sample, and 5 ml of filtrate is used in the test.

$$D \times \frac{V_c}{V_t}$$

$$10 \times \frac{100}{5} = 200$$

$$\frac{100}{\text{Quantity of test sample}}$$

A 1:10 filtrate means that there is 1 ml of serum in 10 ml filtrate; hence, how much serum would be in 5 ml filtrate?

$$\frac{1}{10} = \frac{X}{5}$$

$$10X = 5$$

$$X = 0.5$$

$$\frac{100}{0.5} = 200$$

The same factor, 200, is obtained from both procedures.

The last part of the basic long formula, C_s

$$C_u = \frac{A_u}{A_s} \times C_s$$

$$C_u = \frac{A_u}{A_s} \times \left[W_s \times D \times \frac{V_c}{V_t} \right]$$

has been made into a workable formula.

$$\text{ml std} \times \frac{100}{\text{Quantity of test sample}} \times \text{conc } WS/\text{ml}$$

Be sure the following relationships are understood before continuing:

$$C_u = \frac{A_u}{A_s} \times C_s$$

$$\times W_s \times D \times \frac{V_c}{V_t}$$

$$\times \text{ml std} \times \frac{100}{\text{Quantity of test sample}} \times \text{conc } WS/\text{ml}$$

A colorimetric standard is functionally a solution of known concentration of any substance, which produces a given color of a given intensity under the particular conditions of the test procedure. One may then compare the color produced by a certain quantity of, for example, serum, blood, or urine to that amount of the standard giving the same intensity of color.

EXAMPLE: A sugar procedure used 1 ml of a glucose standard whose concentration is 0.1 mg/ml. The total weight of standard would be 0.1 mg (1×0.1) glucose. The color produced read $50\%T$ (obtained from the instrument reading). If the test sample, 0.5 ml of serum, gave the same color for that particular test procedure, the following is known:

1. 0.1 mg glucose gave a reading of $50\%T$. 2.
2. 0.5 ml serum, under the same conditions, also gave a reading of $50\%T$.

3. Therefore, there must be 0.1 mg glucose in that 0.5 ml of serum.
4. However, the test is not to be reported as glucose per 0.5 ml serum. It is to be reported as glucose per 100 ml serum; hence, use ratio and proportion.

$$\frac{0.1 \text{ mg}}{0.5 \text{ ml}} = \frac{X \text{ mg}}{100 \text{ ml}}$$

$$0.5X = 10$$
$$X = 20 \text{ mg/dl (per 100 ml)}$$

In *this* test procedure, using *this* amount of serum, the color produced by 0.1 mg glucose is equivalent to a blood glucose of 20 mg/dl; hence, this standard, *in this case,* is equivalent to 20 mg/dl. This is the same information that is obtained from the following formula:

$$\left(\text{ml std} \times \frac{100}{\text{Quantity of blood used}}\right) \text{conc of std/ml} = C_s$$

$$\left(1 \times \frac{100}{0.5}\right) 0.1 = C_s$$

$$200 \times 0.1 = C_s$$

$$C_s = 20 \text{ mg/dl}$$

Compare the preceding information with the formula until the relationship between the two is fully understood.

Bear in mind that a given amount of an aqueous standard *will not* always have the same value in different procedures. The value a standard has in any procedure depends on the amount of sample giving the same intensity of color.

EXAMPLE: 1 ml glucose standard (conc/ml = 0.1 mg) is used in each of two procedures. One procedure calls for 0.2 ml serum, and the other uses 0.5 ml serum.

0.2 ml serum	**0.5 ml serum**
1. If 0.2 ml serum gives the same intensity of color as the standard, then, 0.2 ml serum contains 0.1 mg glucose.	2. If 0.5 ml serum gives the same intensity of color as the standard, then, 0.5 ml serum contains 0.1 mg glucose.

$$\frac{0.1 \text{ mg}}{0.2 \text{ ml}} = \frac{X \text{ mg}}{100 \text{ ml}} \qquad\qquad \frac{0.1 \text{ mg}}{0.5 \text{ ml}} = \frac{X \text{ mg}}{100 \text{ ml}}$$

$$0.2X = 10 \qquad\qquad\qquad 0.5X = 10$$
$$X = 50 \qquad\qquad\qquad\quad X = 20$$

1 ml of this standard, *in this procedure,* would equal 50 mg/dl.   1 ml of this standard, *in this procedure,* would equal 20 mg/dl.

Figure this example using the formula

0.2 ml serum	**0.5 ml serum**

$$1 \times \frac{100}{0.2} \times 0.1 = C_s \qquad\qquad 1 \times \frac{100}{0.5} \times 0.1 = C_s$$

$$C_s = 50 \text{ mg/dl} \qquad\qquad\qquad C_s = 20 \text{ mg/dl}$$

The value for any standard in any given procedure is determined by the quantity of serum that produces the same intensity of color under those particular test conditions.

PROCEDURE FOR ESTABLISHING A STANDARD CURVE

There is a general rule that should (in most cases) be followed. When setting up a standard curve, never use more standard, that is, a greater number of milliliters, than the amount of sample (or filtrate) called for in the test procedure. If the test procedure uses 0.5 ml whole blood or serum, then the most standard that should be used is 0.5 ml; if the test procedure uses 3 ml of filtrate, then 3 ml of standard is the most that should be used. The reason for this is to keep the total volume of the test and standard the same.

One exception to the general rule on the volume of standard should be considered. Whenever a very small quantity (such as 0.1 ml or 0.05 ml) of sample, and hence standard, is used and the total volume in the test procedure is relatively large (that is, 10 ml), the addition of another 0.1 ml or so in volume would not really alter the total volume enough to affect it appreciably, and a little extra quantity of standard would be acceptable.

EXAMPLE: Set up a BUN procedure to read from 0 mg/dl to 60 mg/dl. The procedure uses 0.02 ml serum and the only standard available has a concentration of 0.2 mg/ml.

First, calculate the concentration of this standard, for this procedure, in mg/dl.

$$0.02 \times \frac{100}{0.02} \times 0.2 = 20 \text{ mg/dl}$$

The highest point (when one is obeying the general rule) for this standard and in this procedure would be 20 mg/dl.

In this test procedure the following is done: To 0.02 ml serum

1. Add 1 ml reagent *A*
2. Add 1 ml reagent *B*
3. Add 8 ml H_2O

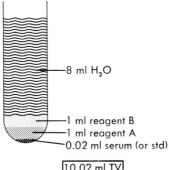

—8 ml H_2O

—1 ml reagent B
—1 ml reagent A
—0.02 ml serum (or std)

10.02 ml TV

If 0.06 ml standard were used in the standard tube instead of the 0.02 ml as before

$$0.06 \times \frac{100}{0.02} \times 0.2 = 60 \text{ mg/dl}$$

—8 ml H_2O

—1 ml reagent B
—1 ml reagent A
—0.06 ml std

10.06 TV

The total volume has been changed from 10.02 ml to 10.06, 0.04 ml, hardly enough to make any difference in the calculations (remember V_u/V_s is omitted when the total volumes are the same). Use common sense when deciding whether or not to follow the general rule.

Consider the following situation:

There is on hand a glucose standard whose concentration on the bottle is stated as

1000 mg/dl. It is to be used in a glucose procedure that uses 5 ml of a 1:20 filtrate solution.

There are several ways to approach the establishment of a standard curve for this procedure. Probably the easiest way would be to decide first (using past experience as a guide) on the highest point needed for the standard. Experience shows that a standard as high as 400 mg/dl could be read on the available instrument when one is using this procedure. Go to the formula and begin to fill it in.

$$\text{ml std} \times \frac{100}{\text{Quantity of sample used}} \times \text{conc of } WS/\text{ml} = C_s$$

Fill in the formula one section at a time.
1. C_s: It was decided that the highest point on the curve should be 400 mg/dl. Therefore, put 400 in place of C_s.
2. ml std: The largest quantity of standard to give this value is required. Since the procedure uses 5 ml filtrate, 5 ml is the largest quantity of standard that one may use following the general rule. Hence, put 5 in place of the ml std.
3. Quantity of sample used: Referring to the procedure, notice that 5 ml of a 1:20 filtrate is used. Since this figure (quantity of sample used) is the *actual amount of blood or serum* (*not* the amount of filtrate), it must be determined how much serum is in the 5 ml of filtrate. A 1:20 filtrate means that there is 1 ml of serum for every 20 ml of filtrate; therefore

$$\frac{1}{20} = \frac{X}{5}$$

$$20X = 5$$
$$X = 0.25 \text{ ml serum in 5 ml filtrate}$$

Put 0.25 in place of quantity of sample used. The problem now stands as follows:

$$\left(5 \times \frac{100}{0.25}\right) X = 400$$

The only information not known is what concentration of standard will yield the value 400 mg/dl; hence, conc of std/ml is the unknown, or X.

$$\left(5 \times \frac{100}{0.25}\right) X = 400$$

$$2000X = 400$$
$$X = 0.2$$

The concentration of the working standard must be 0.2 mg/ml.

To establish a curve at least three points are needed, preferably more. The different points may be determined several ways; one is presented here.

Recall that the total volume of the standard and the unknown (used in the test procedure) should be the same; keep this in mind.

It is known that 5 ml of this particular standard, in this procedure, is equivalent to 400 mg/dl. If less standard is used, it would be equivalent to less milligrams per deciliter. Therefore, fill in the formula using fewer milliliters of standard. Study Fig. 10-1. Take each tube, run each one through the procedure, and read it in the instrument as would be done with the test. The reading taken from the instrument and the corresponding concentrations will now be used to plot the curve.

PLOTTING THE STANDARD CURVE

There are two main types of graph paper generally used in the laboratory: semilog and straight (equal or linear).

$(C_s$ becomes the unknown factor)

Formula

$(4 \times \dfrac{100}{0.25})\ 0.2 = C_s$

$1600 \times 0.2 = 320\ mg/dl$

$(3 \times \dfrac{100}{0.25})\ 0.2 = C_s$

$1200 \times 0.2 = 240\ mg/dl$

$(2 \times \dfrac{100}{0.25})\ 0.2 = C_s$

$800 \times 0.2 = 160\ mg/dl$

A

$(1 \times \dfrac{100}{0.25})\ 0.2 = C_s$

$400 \times 0.2 = 80\ mg/dl$

$(0 \times \dfrac{100}{0.25})\ 0.2 = C_s$

$0 \times 0.2 = 0\ mg/dl$ (blank)

In the test tube

1 ml something (for example, H_2O, saline, or TCA, depending on the test)

4 ml std

5 ml TV (the TV 5 ml must be kept because the test uses 5 ml filtrate)

2 ml liquid

3 ml std

5 ml TV

3 ml liquid

2 ml std
5 ml TV

4 ml liquid

1 ml std
5 ml TV

5 ml liquid

0 ml std ⎫ Blank

5 ml TV ⎭

The following six tubes result.

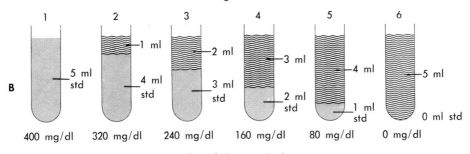

1	2	3	4	5	6
5 ml std	1 ml / 4 ml std	2 ml / 3 ml std	3 ml / 2 ml std	4 ml / 1 ml std	5 ml / 0 ml std
400 mg/dl	320 mg/dl	240 mg/dl	160 mg/dl	80 mg/dl	0 mg/dl

B

Value of the standard

Fig. 10-1

Semilog graph paper (half-log) is exactly what the name implies. The scale for the %T instrument reading is a log scale, and the scale for the concentration values is a straight (linear) scale (Fig. 10-2). *Straight* graph paper has both scales set off in equal units (Fig. 10-3).

These two kinds of graph paper are used because there are two kinds of units of measure on the instruments commonly employed in the laboratory: percent transmittance, %T, and absorbance or optical density, A or OD. Recall that the absorption of light is a logarithmic function and that the absorbance scale is a logarithmic scale that compensates for this. Therefore, absorbance values or readings are usually plotted on straight graph paper because the logarithmic absorption of light has already been taken care of by the A scale. However, the percent transmittance scale is a linear (straight) scale, and when test values are read in %T, there has been no compensation for the logarithmic absorption of light. Hence, %T readings are usually plotted on semilog paper, as this would correct for the logarithmic function.

Either type reading may be plotted on either type graph paper; however, consider the following: to see if a straight line is formed, that is, Beer's law followed, absorbance must be plotted on straight paper and %T on semilog paper. If there is no desire to know whether Beer's law is followed and the proper paper is not available, use the other type. It is easier and a little more accurate to read values from a straight curve rather than one that is not straight, but it is by no means mandatory. Do not decide against using

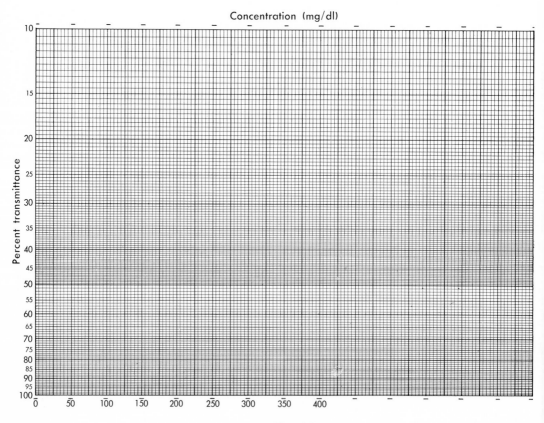

Fig. 10-2

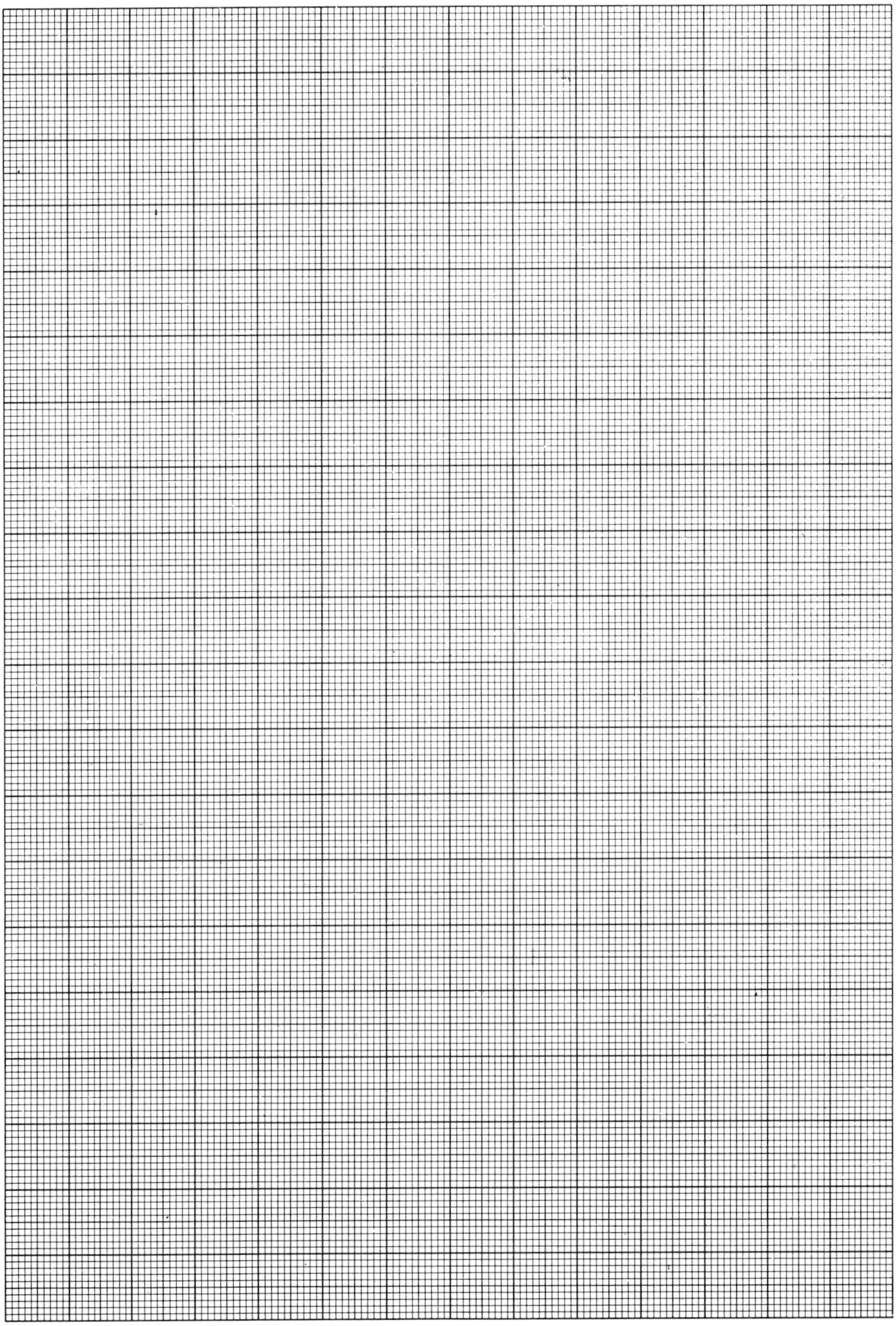

Fig. 10-3

a curve just because the correct paper is not available. Simply be sure the limitations are clearly understood!

CAUTION: Never draw the lines of the curve past the last point on the curve! What happens to the relationship between the readings and the concentration is not known beyond the extremes of the curve. Also, values as low as 10 (in %T readings) should not be used in actual practice. It is used here for convenience and simplicity.

Using the values from the glucose problem earlier and the %T and A values given below, plot a curve each of the four possible ways (see the following).

Standard value	%T readings	A readings
400 mg/dl	10	1.0
320 mg/dl	16	0.8
240 mg/dl	25	0.6
160 mg/dl	39.5	0.4
80 mg/dl	63	0.2
0 mg/dl (reagent blank)	100	0.0

Notice here the percent transmittance, %T, readings and the absorbance, A, readings in relation to the concentration of the standard. Recall that absorbance is directly related to the concentration. Notice that the absorbance reading that corresponds to 80 mg/dl is 0.2. As the concentration doubles (to 160 mg/dl) the absorbance doubles (to 0.4 A). When the concentration is four times greater ($80 \times 4 = 320$ mg/dl), the absorbance is four times greater ($4 \times 0.2 = 0.8$). However, no such relationship exists between the %T readings and the concentration, for there has been no adjustment for the logarithmic relationship of the absorption of light by the substance.

The four types of plots to make are shown in Figs. 10-4 to 10-7 (first on the correct paper, then on the opposite paper). Consider the following:

Fig. 10-4: With absorbance readings plotted on straight paper, it is evident that Beer's law is followed.

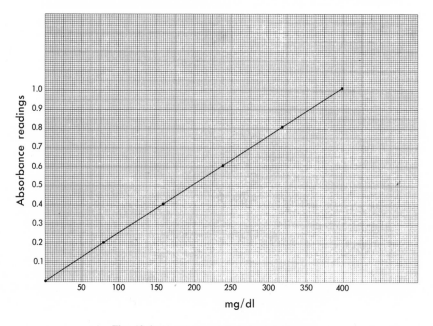

Fig. 10-4. Absorbance plotted on straight paper.

Fig. 10-5: With %*T* readings plotted on semilog paper, it is evident that Beer's law is followed.

Fig. 10-6: With absorbance readings plotted on semilog paper, it is not known whether the curve develops because of the semilog paper or because the procedure does not follow Beer's law.

Fig. 10-7: With %*T* readings plotted on straight paper, it is not known if the curve develops because of the straight paper or because the procedure does not follow Beer's law.

If readings are taken from each curve, the following values result (Fig. 10-4 through 10-7):

Sample instrument reading			Value from curve used			
No.	%*T*	*A*	%*T* (semilog)	%*T* (straight)	*A* (semilog)	*A* (straight)
1.	50	0.3	120 mg/dl	120 mg/dl	120 mg/dl	120 mg/dl
2.	80	0.097	38 mg/dl	37 mg/dl	42 mg/dl	38 mg/dl
3.	30	0.52	208 mg/dl	208 mg/dl	208 mg/dl	208 mg/dl

Essentially, the same answer is obtained from each curve. Those plotted on the correct paper are just a little easier to read and also give some information about Beer's law.

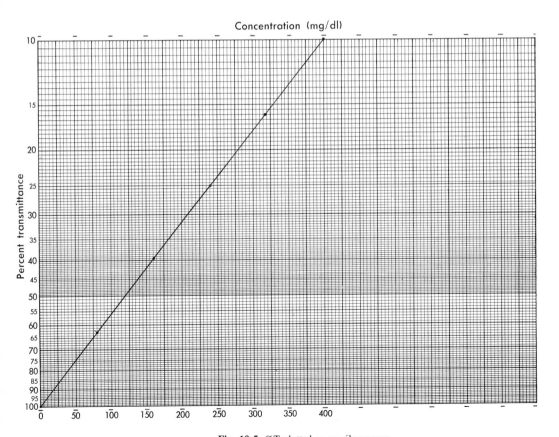

Fig. 10-5. %T plotted on semilog paper.

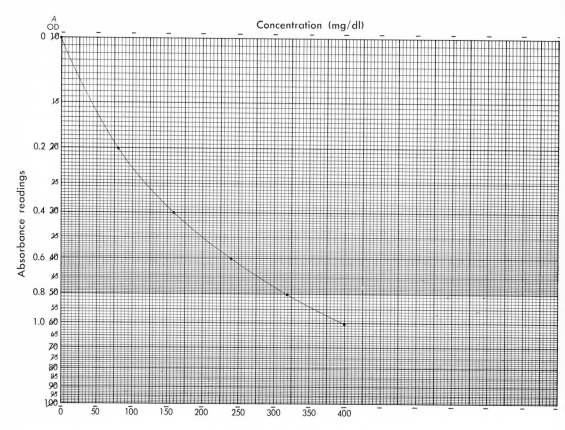

Fig. 10-6. Absorbance plotted on semilog paper.

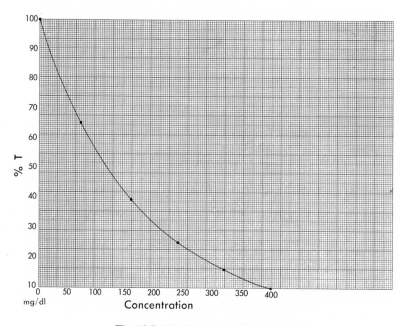

Fig. 10-7. %T plotted on straight paper.

USE OF REFERENCE (BLANK) SOLUTIONS

Most colorimetric procedures use some kind of reference solution to calibrate the colorimeter for the particular test solution used. These reference solutions are usually referred to as blank solutions. The most convenient, common type of blank solution is the reagent blank. This solution contains the same concentration of all the reagents used in the preparation of the standard and test solutions. However, it does not contain any of the substance for which the test is being made.

When a reagent blank is put into a colorimeter any response is due to factors other than the test substance. The machine is then set on $100\%T$ or $0\ A$. These values are used to represent zero concentration, and any response of the machine would be due to the substance for which the test is being made.

In some test procedures a specialized reference solution may be used to modify the colorimeter readings. In many of these procedures the instrument is set at $0\ A$ or $100\%T$ using only distilled water as a blank. In such cases the reading of the test solution must be adjusted using the reading of the specialized blank solution.

In these procedures there is one common pitfall in the adjustment of the readings. One must not use the percent transmittance scale without the proper consideration of the logarithmic absorption of light by substances. This mistake is made frequently in the clinical laboratory.

There are several ways the colorimetric readings may be corrected using the specialized blank solution. Three will be considered here.

One method commonly used is to mentally move the reading of the specialized blank down the scale to $0\ A$ or $100\%T$. The readings of the standard or test solutions are moved a corresponding number of units down the scale. This procedure will produce accurate results with the absorbance scale. It will *not* make a proper adjustment of the percent transmittance readings.

EXAMPLE: A test was made using a procedure directing that the colorimeter be adjusted to $0\ A$ or $100\%T$ using distilled water for the blank solution. A specialized blank was used to compare with the test solution. The absorbance of the specialized blank was 0.1 and the absorbance of the test was 0.5. The test reading can be adjusted by mentally moving the reading down the scale 0.1 A units, so that the absorbance reading of the specialized blank can be thought of as $0\ A$. The test reading is then mentally moved the same number of units down the scale and will now be 0.4 A (note Fig. 10-8).

If this same general procedure were done using the percent transmittance scale, the test reading would be incorrect (study Fig. 10-9). The corresponding percent transmittance of the specialized blank is 79.5 and the percent transmittance of the test is 31.5. If the readings are moved down the scale 20.5 units, so that the specialized blank is at $100\%T$, then the test reading would be at 52. This is *not* equal to 0.4 A.

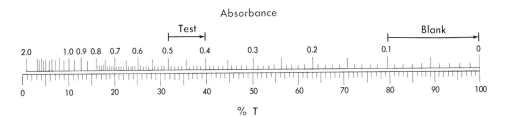

Fig. 10-8

Absorbance

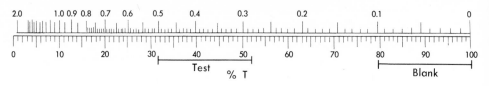

Fig. 10-9

Another method of adjusting a test reading with a specialized blank is to subtract the smaller reading from the larger. Again, this will work for the absorbance scale, but it will *not* work for percent transmittance. Consider the values from the preceding example.

Absorbance	Percent transmittance
0.5	79.5
0.1	31.5
0.4	48.0

A third method would be to take the concentration value of the specialized blank and the test solution from the standard curve. The value for the specialized blank is then subtracted from the value for the test. This method will work for readings taken as absorbance or percent transmittance (study Table 7). Note the final concentration values when absorbance and percent transmittance are used in these three ways.

Note that the same answer is obtained for the test values using absorbance (*A* or *OD*) readings all three ways. This is true for two main reasons: (1) absorbance is *directly* related to concentration and (2) the logarithmic absorption of light is taken care of at the time of reading.

However, notice that the only way to obtain the correct answer (160 mg/dl) using percent transmittance readings is to get the values from the percent transmittance curve and then to subtract the blank value from the test value. The reason for this being that until the readings have been taken from the curve there has been no correction for the logarithmic absorption of light, and percent transmittance readings are *not* directly related to concentration.

Study the preceding relationships until they are thoroughly understood.

Table 7

	Value from the appropriate curve	
Procedure	**%T curve** (Fig. 10-5)	***A* curve** (Fig. 10-4)
1. Move down the scale and read. $\quad$0.5 → 0.1 = 0.4; A = 0.4 $\quad$31.5 → 20.5 = 52; $\%T$ = 52	113 mg/dl	160 mg/dl
2. Subtract readings. $\quad A$ = 0.5 − 0.1 = 0.4 $\quad \%T$ = 79.5 − 31.5 = 48	126 mg/dl	160 mg/dl
3. Read values from curve; subtract values. $\quad A$ = 0.5; 0.1 $\quad \%T$ = 31.5; 79.5	31.5 = 200 79.5 = $\underline{\quad 40}$ 160 mg/dl	0.5 = 200 0.1 = $\underline{\quad 40}$ 160 mg/dl

SERUM STANDARDS

The aqueous standards discussed previously are not always treated exactly as the sample all the way through the procedure. For this reason the value (concentration) given on the aqueous standard bottle may or may not be the equivalent concentration for the standard in that particular procedure. The same standard may be equivalent to more than one sample concentration, depending on the procedure used.

Serum standards, on the other hand, are usually treated exactly as the test sample, all the way through the procedure. For this reason the concentration on the bottle usually is the equivalent concentration for that procedure, and the concentration for a serum standard will usually be the same no matter what procedure it is used in.

EXAMPLE: Consider a serum standard for glucose. Concentration 100 mg/dl is stated on the bottle; therefore, the value expected for this standard when it is used in a procedure is 100 mg/dl. Use this same standard in two different glucose procedures.

1. This procedure used 5 ml of a 1:10 filtrate.   2. This procedure used 3 ml of a 1:20 filtrate.

std = 100 mg/dl
std = 100 mg/100 ml
std = 1 mg/ml

A 1:10 filtrate = 1 ml serum/10 ml filtrate.

$$\frac{1}{10} = \frac{X}{5}$$

$$10X = 5$$
$$X = 0.5 \text{ ml serum/5 ml filtrate}$$

$$\text{ml std} \times \frac{100}{0.5} \times 1 = C_s$$

std = 100 mg/dl
std = 100 mg/100 ml
std = 1 mg/ml

A 1:20 filtrate = 1 ml serum/20 ml filtrate.

$$\frac{1}{20} = \frac{X}{3}$$

$$20X = 3$$
$$X = 0.15 \text{ ml serum/3 ml filtrate}$$

$$\text{ml std} \times \frac{100}{0.15} \times 1 = C_s$$

The information missing in the last expression of each preceding method is the number of milliliters of standard used. This is the thing making serum standards different in calculations from aqueous standards. Since serum standards are treated *exactly* as the unknowns, a filtrate is made of them also. And since the *ml std* means the number of milliliters of *actual* standard (not filtrate), one must calculate the amount of standard present in the quantity of filtrate used.

EXAMPLE: Consider the standard for the two preceding procedures.

1. 1:10 filtrate = 1 ml std/10 ml filtrate.   2. 1:20 filtrate = 1 ml std/20 ml filtrate.

$$\frac{1}{10} = \frac{X}{5}$$

$$10X = 5$$
$$X = 0.5 \text{ ml std/5 ml filtrate}$$

$$\frac{1}{20} = \frac{X}{3}$$

$$20X = 3$$
$$X = 0.15 \text{ ml std/3 ml filtrate}$$

therefore

$$0.5 \times \frac{100}{0.5} \times 1 = C_s$$

$$C_s = 100 \text{ mg/dl}$$

$$0.15 \times \frac{100}{0.15} \times 1 = C_s$$

$$C_s = 100 \text{ mg/dl}$$

Think carefully about these examples and be sure the principles are understood before continuing.

In some instances, a substance needed for a standard is not available, for one reason or another, in pure form. In this case, a compound is used that contains this specific substance but that also contains other substances. For example, if a nitrogen standard is needed, $(NH_4)_2SO_4$ may be used. Figure out how much of the compound used would contain the quantity of nitrogen desired.

EXAMPLE: Make a 4 mg/dl nitrogen standard using $(NH_4)_2SO_4$.

The molecular weight of $(NH_4)_2SO_4$ is 132; the molecular weight of nitrogen is 14; there are 2 atoms of nitrogen in the compound; hence, there would be 28 mg of nitrogen in every 132 mg $(NH_4)_2SO_4$. If 100 ml of this standard is to be made, 4 mg of nitrogen would be needed.

$$\frac{28N}{132} = \frac{4N}{X}$$

$$28X = 528$$
$$X = 18.86 \text{ mg } (NH_4)_2SO_4 \text{ (contains 4 mg nitrogen)}$$

Therefore, dilute 18.86 gm $(NH_4)_2SO_4$ up to 100 ml to yield a nitrogen standard whose concentration is 4 mg N/dl.

Practice problems

1. How much $(NH_4)_2SO_4$ would be needed to make a nitrogen standard with a concentration of 10 mg N/dl?
2. A stock standard is available; stated on the label is a concentration of 1000 mg/dl. How would 50 ml of a 0.5 mg/dl working standard be prepared?
3. A certain procedure says to use 5 ml of a 1:20 filtrate. What concentration of working standard would be needed to set up a curve whose highest point was 400 mg/dl?
4. How would the working standard for problem 3 be made from a stock standard whose concentration was 200 mg/dl?
5. In a procedure that uses 0.02 ml serum in the test, what would be the value of a standard whose concentration was 10 mg/dl?
6. A new glucose curve is needed. The usual readable range is 0 to 350 mg/dl. The procedure uses 0.3 ml of a 1:10 filtrate. The concentration of the stock standard is 50 mg/100 ml.
   a. What is the highest point that can be made for the curve?
   b. How much standard *(WS)* will be used to give this point?
   c. What concentration of *WS* will be needed?
   d. How will this be made from the *SS*?
   e. What other points will there be on the curve, and how will they be arrived at (show formulas and work)?
7. In a Chloride procedure (which uses 5 ml of a 1:10 filtrate) 5 ml of 0.06N $Hg(NO_3)_2$ are used to titrate 5 ml of the filtrate. What is the Chloride concentration in mEq/l and in mg/dl?
8. In a Kjeldahl assay, 1.0 ml of 0.2N HCl are needed for titration. What is the nitrogen content in the sample?
9. If the sample in problem 8 had been 5 ml serum, what would the nitrogen content be in mEq/l and in mg/dl (eq wt N = 14)?
10. If 2 ml of 0.005N $KMnO_4$ (eq wt = 31) are required to titrate the calcium in a 2 ml aliquot of serum, what is the calcium concentration in mg/dl?

CHAPTER 11

Hematology math

There are two main areas in hematology that have some mathematics connected with them: (1) the dilution of blood in the RBC and WBC pipettes and the counting chamber and (2) the indices.

It is true that, today, the majority of laboratories make cell counts on particle counters. But even so, there will be times when the laboratory worker will need to be able to use, and compute the results using, a counting chamber and the pipettes.

PIPETTES

The pipettes used in hematology are composed of two main parts: (1) a stem, sub-divided into two (or sometimes ten) equal parts and (2) a bulb containing a bead, which serves three purposes: (a) to identify (white or clear bead for a WBC pipette and a red bead for the RBC pipette), (b) to aid in mixing when the pipette is full or partially full, and (c) to indicate dryness when the pipette is empty and clean.

The dilutions used in these calculations are based on the fact that the volume of the bulb is ten times the volume of the stem in the WBC pipette and 100 times the volume of the stem in the RBC pipette. Since the blood in the stem is drawn up into the bulb for dilution and since the total volume of the bulb is 10 for the WBC pipettes and 100 for the RBC pipettes, the denominators for the WBC and the RBC dilutions are always 10 and 100, respectively (study Fig. 11-1).

Notice the WBC pipette in Figure 11-1. There are 11 total parts (or volumes) from the tip of the stem to the 11 mark. There is 1 volume from the tip to the 1 mark, and there are 10 volumes from the 1 mark to the 11 mark. Since the diluting fluid remaining in the stem (1 part) does not take part in the dilution, the total volume for the dilution process is 10 parts (11 total parts minus 1 part in the stem). If the blood had been drawn up to the 0.5 mark in a WBC pipette and diluted up to the 11 mark with diluting fluid, there would be 0.5 parts of blood in a total volume of 10 parts: a 0.5/10 dilution.

Remember, for ease of understanding and to have a factor that is easy to work with, one usually expresses a dilution as a 1-to-something dilution; therefore

$$\frac{0.5}{10} = \frac{1}{X}$$
$$0.5X = 10$$
$$X = 20$$
$$1/20 \text{ dilution}$$

Recall that to correct for a dilution, one must multiply by the reciprocal. Hence, the dilution factor for blood drawn to the 0.5 mark in a WBC pipette is 20 (the reciprocal of $1/20$).

Now look at the RBC pipette in Fig. 11-1. The stem has a smaller bore, and the bulb is larger. The total number of parts from the tip of the stem to the 101 mark is 101 total parts, but, again, because the 1 part of fluid remaining in the stem does not enter into the dilution, the total parts for diluting purposes are 100 (101 total parts − 1 part in the

121

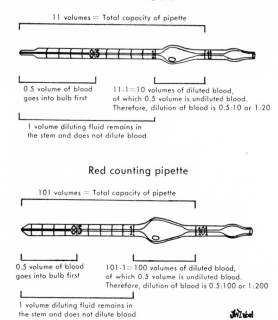

White counting pipette

11 volumes = Total capacity of pipette

0.5 volume of blood goes into bulb first

11-1=10 volumes of diluted blood, of which 0.5 volume is undiluted blood. Therefore, dilution of blood is 0.5:10 or 1:20

1 volume diluting fluid remains in the stem and does not dilute blood

Red counting pipette

101 volumes = Total capacity of pipette

0.5 volume of blood goes into bulb first

101-1=100 volumes of diluted blood, of which 0.5 volume is undiluted blood. Therefore, dilution of blood is 0.5:100 or 1:200

1 volume diluting fluid remains in the stem and does not dilute blood

Fig. 11-1. Explanation of dilution of blood in red and white cell counting pipettes. (From Bauer, J. D., Ackermann, P. G., and Toro, G.: Clinical laboratory methods, ed. 8, St. Louis, 1974, The C. V. Mosby Co.)

stem = 100 parts). If the blood were drawn to the 0.5 mark in a RBC pipette and diluted up to the 101 mark, the dilution would be

$$\frac{0.5}{100} = \frac{1}{X}$$

$$0.5X = 100$$
$$X = 200$$
$$1/200 \text{ dilution}$$
$$\text{Dilution factor} = 200$$

EXAMPLES: What would the dilution and the dilution factor be in the following instances?

1. In a WBC pipette the blood is drawn to the 0.4 mark.

$$\frac{0.4}{10} = \frac{1}{X}$$

$$0.4X = 10$$
$$X = 25$$
$$1/25 \text{ dilution}$$
$$\text{Dilution factor} = 25$$

2. In a RBC pipette the blood is drawn to the 0.2 mark.

$$\frac{0.2}{100} = \frac{1}{X}$$

$$0.2X = 100$$
$$X = 500$$
$$1/500 \text{ dilution}$$
$$\text{Dilution factor} = 500$$

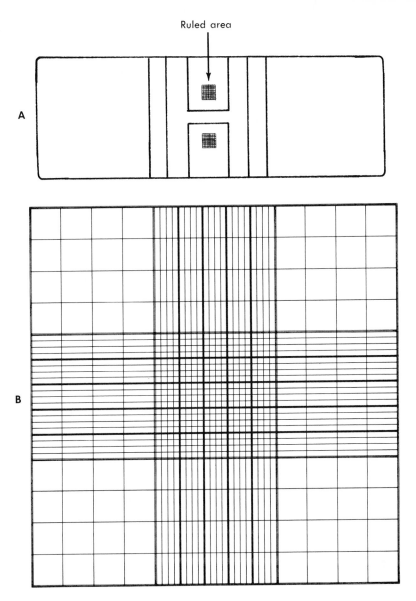

Fig. 11-2. Area for counting cells.

COUNTING CHAMBER

There are three dimensions of the counting chamber with which one should be thoroughly familiar.

1. Length = one dimension = millimeters (in this case) = mm
2. Area = two dimensions = length × width = square millimeters = mm^2
3. Volume = three dimensions = length × width × height (depth) = cubic millimeters = mm^3

Red and white cell counts are reported as the number of cells/mm^3. (A cubic millimeter is a very minute quantity. Assuming 60 drops/ml, a cubic millimeter is approximately $1/16$ of a drop.)

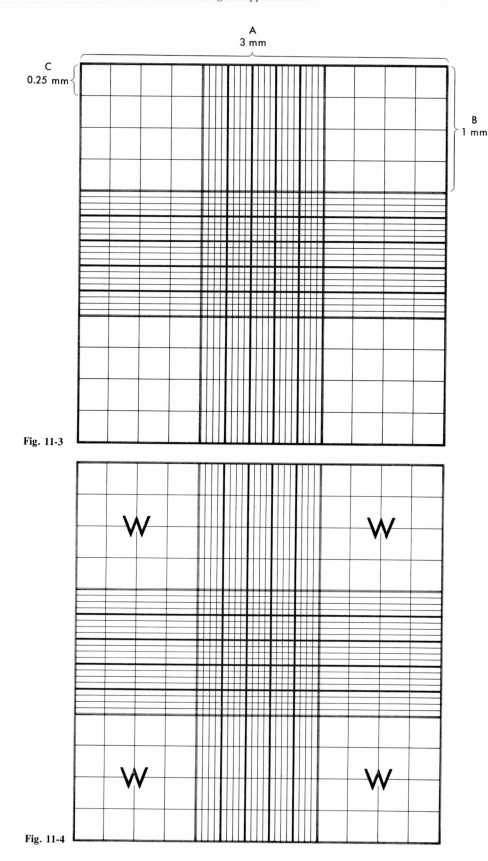

Fig. 11-3

Fig. 11-4

The counting chamber is used for performing red and white blood counts. The ruled area (Fig. 11-2, *A*) is presented enlarged in Fig. 11-2, *B*. Examine it closely.

Notice that the entire length of the ruled area is 3 mm (Fig. 11-3, *A*). That means that the *entire* area of one ruled area (on one side on the counting chamber) is 9 mm² (area = L × W; 3 × 3 = 9 mm²). The entire ruled area is composed of nine squares, each 1 mm². The length of the sides of these largest squares is 1 mm; 1 × 1 = 1 mm² (Fig. 11-3, *B*). These squares (1 mm²) are referred to as *white* squares, because the four corner squares, Fig. 11-4, are usually used for the white blood count.

These white squares are further divided into 16 smaller squares, Fig. 11-3, *C*, whose sides are 0.25 mm in length (1 mm ÷ 4 = 0.25; there are four divisions on that 1 mm).

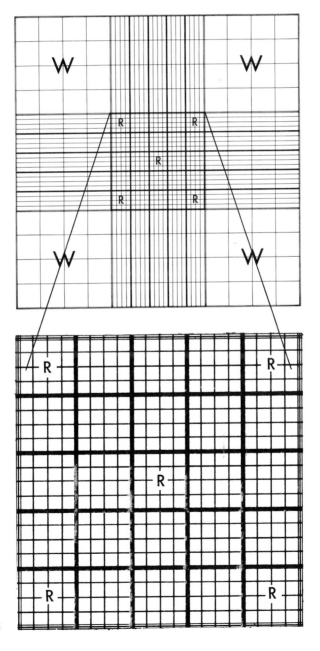

Fig. 11-5

The central square mm (Fig. 11-5) is subdivided into 25 squares, sometimes referred to as *red squares*. The four corner squares and the central square are usually used to perform the red blood count. Each of these 25 squares (Fig. 11-6, *A*) are subdivided into 16 smaller squares (Fig. 11-6, *B*). The length of *A* is 0.2 mm (1 ÷ 5 = 0.2). The length of *B* is 0.05 mm (0.2 ÷ 4 = 0.05).

It seems confusing at first, but try to remember two main things: (1) the length of each of the nine large squares is 1 mm and (2) the squares are subdivided—16, 25, and 16 (the white squares into 16, the middle square into 25, and each of the 25 into 16). Remembering this, the length of any line and the area of any square can always be figured out (not memorized).

Examine Fig. 11-7. Most counting chambers (certain ones for special purposes may be different) are made so that the center platform, *A*, which bears the ruled areas, is exactly 0.1 mm lower than the raised side ridges, *B*, which support the cover slip, *C*. It is into this space, *D*, between the cover slip and this center platform that the diluted blood, which is to be counted, flows. Therefore, the depth of the fluid being counted is 0.1 mm.

There are three factors to be considered when calculating the results obtained from the use of the pipettes and counting chamber: (1) pertains to the pipettes and (2) and (3) pertain to the counting chamber.

1. Whole blood was not used, therefore, a *dilution factor* is needed.
2. The counts are reported in the number of cells/mm³. If one could count a space 1 mm × 1 mm × 1 mm, one would have 1 mm³.

$$\underbrace{1 \text{ mm} \times 1 \text{ mm}}_{\text{area}} \times \underbrace{1 \text{ mm}}_{\text{depth}} = 1 \text{ mm}^3$$

But the depth is 0.1 mm, not 1 mm ($^1/_{10}$ what it should be); therefore a *depth factor*

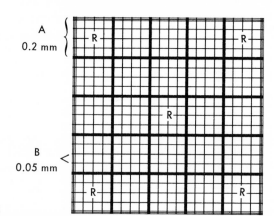

Fig. 11-6

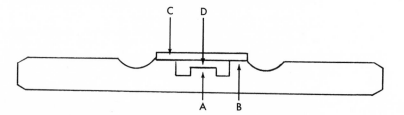

Fig. 11-7

(10) is needed to correct for this. Unless stated otherwise, the depth factor for problems presented here will always be 10.

3. Area counted. If 1 mm² were counted, an *area factor* would not be needed. If more or less than 1 mm² is counted, this should be corrected for. Use 1/area counted (in mm²) for determining the area factor (recall: divide by what was used and multiply by what should have been used). Notice the area counted in mm² and the area factor *are not* the same thing.

Using these three factors, one obtains the following basic formula:

$$\text{Depth factor} \times \text{Area factor} \times \text{Dilution factor} = \text{Final factor}$$

$$\text{Final factor} \times \text{Cells counted (in the area used for the area factor)} = \text{Cells/mm}^3$$

If the area factor is expanded, the following formula develops:

$$\text{Depth factor} \times \frac{1}{\text{Area counted in mm}^2} \times \text{Dilution factor} = \text{Final factor}$$

Then combine; the formula becomes

$$\frac{\text{Depth factor} \times \text{Dilution factor}}{\text{Area counted in mm}^2 \text{ (not area factor)}} = \text{Final factor}$$

There is one other factor that may, at times, be seen. Some authors refer to a *volume correction factor* (or volume factor). Since volume is $L \times W \times H$, the factor may be arrived at in the following two ways:

1. The volume that should be counted is 1 mm³. Using the rule, divide by what was used and multiply by what should have been used, one may find the volume factor by 1/volume counted. Divide by the volume actually counted (length of area counted × width of area counted × depth = volume in mm³; or since $L \times W$ is area; area × depth = volume in mm³) and multiply by 1 (the 1 mm³, which should have been counted). Again, notice that the volume counted and the volume factor are not the same thing.

2. One may multiply the *area factor,* not area counted, times the *depth factor* to obtain the volume factor.

The formula presented earlier for calculating the final factor may be expressed in several ways. Four other expressions of this formula are presented below. Understand the relationships and the fact that they are all different expressions of the same thing before continuing!

$$\text{Dilution factor} \times \text{Depth factor} \times \frac{1}{\text{Area counted}} = \text{Final factor}$$

$$\text{Dilution factor} \times \text{Depth factor} \times \text{Area factor} = \text{Final factor}$$

$$\text{Dilution factor} \times \frac{1}{\text{Volume counted}} = \text{Final factor}$$

$$\text{Dilution factor} \times \text{Volume factor} = \text{Final factor}$$

In everyday practice, use the one that seems easiest for you.

Study the following examples, and give the following information for each:

A. Dilution of blood   E. Volume factor (determined two ways)

B. Dilution factor   F. Final factor

C. Depth factor   G. Cells/mm³

D. Area factor (expressed two ways)

EXAMPLE: In a WBC pipette the blood is drawn to the 0.8 mark. Six *white* squares are counted. 100 cells are counted.

A. Dilution:

$$\frac{0.8}{10} = \frac{1}{X}$$

$$0.8X = 10$$
$$X = 12.5$$
$$1/12.5 \text{ dilution}$$

B. Dilution factor: Reciprocal of $1/12.5 = 12.5$.

C. Depth factor: Since no information was given concerning the counting chamber depth, assume a standard counting chamber with a depth of 0.1 mm. This is $1/10$ of 1 mm, so the depth factor is 10.

D. Area factor:

$$\frac{1}{\text{Area counted in mm}^2}$$

One has been asked to count six *white* squares. A white square is one of the nine larger squares, each 1 mm². Therefore, if six of them are counted, six mm² have been counted. Hence, the area factor may be either of the following:

1.

$$\frac{1}{\text{Area counted in mm}^2}$$

$$\frac{1}{6} \text{ (left as a fraction)}$$

2.

$$\frac{1}{\text{Area counted in mm}^2}$$

$$\frac{1}{6} = 0.167$$

E. Volume factor: Determined two ways

1. Volume factor $= \dfrac{1}{\text{Volume counted}}$

$L \times W \times H = \text{Volume in mm}^3$

The squares counted would not be lined up as below on the counting chamber; they are presented this way so the length and width can be easily figured. If 6 mm² were counted, the L and W would be

6mm

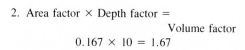

$\}$ 1 mm

$L = 6$ mm, $W = 1$ mm, $H = 0.1$
$6 \times 1 \times 0.1 = 0.6$ mm³ counted
$1/0.6$ or $1.67 = $ Volume factor

2. Area factor $\times$ Depth factor $=$

Volume factor

$0.167 \times 10 = 1.67$

F. Final factor:

1. $\dfrac{\text{Depth factor} \times \text{Dilution factor}}{\text{Area counted in mm}^2} = \text{Final factor}$

$$\frac{10 \times 12.5}{6} = 20.8$$

2. Depth factor $\times$ Area factor $\times$ Dilution factor $=$ Final factor

$$10 \times 0.167 \times 12.5 = 20.8$$

3. Volume factor $\times$ Dilution factor $=$ Final factor

$$1.67 \times 12.5 = 20.8$$

G. Cells/mm³:

$$\text{Cells counted} \times \text{Final factor} = \text{Cells/mm}^3$$

$$100 \times 20.8 = 2080 \text{ cells/mm}^3$$

EXAMPLE: In a RBC pipette the blood is diluted to the 0.2 mark. Five *red* squares are counted. A counting chamber with a depth of 0.2mm was used. 150 cells were counted.

A. Dilution:

$$\frac{0.2}{100} = \frac{1}{X}$$

$$0.2X = 100$$

$$X = 500$$

$$1/500 \text{ dilution}$$

B. Dilution factor: Reciprocal of $^1/_{500}$ is 500.

C. Depth factor: 0.2 mm is $^1/_5$ the depth that should have been counted. Therefore, the depth factor is 5.

$$\frac{1}{0.2} \text{ or } 5$$

D. Area factor: The central square used for red counts is 1 mm², subdivided into 25 smaller squares, each of which is $^1/_{25}$ mm². If five of these smaller squares were counted, $^5/_{25} = ^1/_5 = 0.2$ mm² (area counted in mm²) would have been counted (1/0.2 or 5).

E. Volume factor:

$$1.0 \times 0.2 \times 0.2 = 0.04 \text{ mm}^3 \qquad \text{Depth factor} \times \text{Area Factor} = \text{Volume factor}$$

$$\frac{1}{0.04} = 25 \qquad\qquad 5 \times 5 = 25$$

F. Final factor:

$$\frac{5 \times 500}{0.2} = 12{,}500$$

G. Cells counted/mm³: $150 \times 12{,}500 = 1{,}875{,}000$ cells/mm³.

Sometimes it is necessary to correct a white count if there are many nucleated red blood cells (NRBC) present. This is because the white cell diluting fluids and the substances used in electronic counting procedures lyse the red cells as usual, but the nucleus (which is not usually present) remains and is counted as a white cell.

There are several ways to correct this for extra counting. The method presented below does not rely on memorization. It is a ratio-proportion setup.

	Differential	**Counting chamber**
Actual count (WBC only)	$\dfrac{100}{100 + \text{NRBC}/100 \text{ WBC}}$	$= \dfrac{X}{\text{WBC counted}}$
Combined count (WBC + NRBC)		

Look at the preceding formula. There are two ratios. The one on the left pertains to the differential; the one on the right pertains to the counting chamber. The top figure in each ratio is the number of *actual* white cells (the 100 is the actual number of white cells counted on the differential, and X is the true white count, which is the figure desired). The bottom numbers in each ratio are the combined counts, white cells plus nucleated red blood cells (the 100 + NRBC is the number of white cells counted on the differential, 100, plus the number of NRBC present along with that 100 white cells). The *WBC counted* is the number of white blood cells counted by whatever method was used. This count includes both white cells and the nucleus of the NRBC.

EXAMPLE: A white count of 25,000 is obtained. When the differential was performed, 100 white cells were counted, and along with these 100 white cells, 50 NRBC were seen. That means there were 150 cells counted, 100 of which were white cells. Using this information, fill in the ratio and proportion. If there are 100 WBC in every 150 cells, then there will be X WBC in 25,000 cells.

$$\frac{100}{150} = \frac{X}{25,000}$$

$$150X = 2,500,000$$
$$X = 16,667$$

The actual white count is $16,667/mm^3$.

INDICES

There are three mean corpuscular values (indices) that are commonly calculated. They are
1. Mean corpuscular volume (MCV)
2. Mean corpuscular hemoglobin (MCH)
3. Mean corpuscular hemoglobin concentration (MCHC)

These values are concerned with the volume of the average erythrocyte and the amount of hemoglobin in the average erythrocyte.

For all of the examples presented here, the following values will be used: hemoglobin (Hb), 15 gm%; hematocrit (Hct), 50%; red blood cell (RBC) count, 5,000,000.

Mean corpuscular volume

The mean corpuscular volume is the *volume* of the average erythrocyte. Normal values lie between 80 to 90 μm^3 (cubic because it concerns volume).

The following formula is used to calculate the mean corpuscular volume:

$$MCV = \frac{Hct \times 10}{RBC \text{ (in millions)}} \qquad \text{(formula 1)}$$

Since the mean corpuscular volume is the volume (in cubic microns) of the average erythrocyte, if the number of cubic microns of cells in 1 mm^3 are known and that number is divided by the number of cells per cubic millimeter, the volume (in cubic microns) of one erythrocyte would be known. Therefore

$$MCV = \frac{Cubic \text{ microns of cells in 1 } mm^3 \text{ of blood}}{Cells/mm^3 \text{ of blood}} \qquad \text{(formula 2)}$$

To find the number of cubic microns of cells/mm^3 of blood, the numerator, one needs to know the following:

1. How many cubic microns = 1 mm^3?

$$1 \text{ mm} \times 1 \text{ mm} \times 1 \text{ mm} = 1 \text{ mm}^3$$
$$1 \text{ mm} = 1000\mu$$
$$1000 \ \mu m \times 1000 \ \mu m \times 1000 \ \mu m = 1,000,000,000 \ \mu m^3$$
$$1 \text{ mm}^3 = 10^9 \ \mu m^3$$

Hence, 1 mm^3 of blood equals 10^9 μm^3 of blood

2. How much of the 10^9 μm^3 of blood is cells? The hematocrit determines what percentage of blood is erythrocytes; therefore, multiply 10^9 μm^3 by the hematocrit to find out how much of the blood is erythrocytes.

$$10^9 \times 0.50$$

The cells/mm³ of blood, the denominator, has been given as 5,000,000 (5×10^6) cells/mm³. Hence

$$MCV = \frac{10^9 \times 0.50}{5 \times 10^6} \qquad \text{(step 1)}$$

$$MCV = \frac{0.50 \times 10^9}{5 \times 10^6} \qquad \text{(step 2)}$$

$$MCV = \frac{0.50 \times 10^{9-6}}{5} \qquad \text{(step 3)}$$

$$MCV = \frac{0.50 \times 10^3}{5} \qquad \text{(step 4)}$$

$$MCV = \frac{0.50 \times 1000}{5} \qquad \text{(step 5)}$$

$$MCV = \frac{500}{5} \qquad \text{(step 6)}$$

$$MCV = 100 \ \mu m^3 \qquad \text{(step 7)}$$

Look at step 6.

$$MCV = \frac{500}{5} = \frac{50 \ (Hct) \times 10}{5 \ (RBC \ in \ millions)} = \frac{500}{5} = 100 \ \mu m^3$$

The preceding steps 1 through 7 and formula 2 are what the calculations for the mean corpuscule volume are actually based on, but since the numbers representing the hematocrit and RBC (in millions) give the same answer and are much easier to work in daily calculations, formula 1 is the one usually given. However, one should know what it represents.

Mean corpuscular hemoglobin

The mean corpuscular hemoglobin is the *weight* of hemoglobin in the average erythrocyte. Normal values lie between 27 and 32 micromicrograms (written $\mu\mu g$ or pg, picograms, *grams* because of *weight*). The following formula is used to calculate the mean corpuscular hemoglobin:

$$MCH = \frac{Hb \ in \ grams \times 10}{RBC \ (in \ millions)} \qquad \text{(formula 3)}$$

Mean corpuscular hemoglobin is the weight of hemoglobin in the average red blood cell. If the number of picograms in 1 mm³ of blood is known and that number is divided by the number of red cells in 1 mm³ of blood, the number of picograms of hemoglobin per erythrocyte will be known.

$$MCH = \frac{pg \ hemoglobin/mm^3 \ of \ blood}{Cells/mm^3} \qquad \text{(formula 4)}$$

To find pg hemoglobin/mm³ of blood, the numerator, convert the patient's hemoglobin value/100 ml of blood to picograms of hemoglobin per cubic millimeter of blood.

$$1 \ gm = 10^{12} \ picograms$$
$$1 \ ml = 1 \ cm^3$$
$$1 \ cm \times 1 \ cm \times 1 \ cm = 1 \ cm^3$$
$$1 \ cm = 10 \ mm$$
$$10 \ mm \times 10 \ mm \times 10 \ mm = 1000 \ mm^3$$

Hence, 1 ml = 1000 mm^3.

For example, 15 gm/100 ml converted to pg/mm^3 =

$$\frac{gm \times 10^{12}}{ml \times 10^3} = \frac{15 \times 10^{12}}{100 \times 10^3} = 15 \times 10^7 \text{ pg hemoglobin/mm}^3 \text{ of blood (the numerator)}$$

The cells/mm^3 of blood, the denominator, has been given as 5,000,000 (5 × 10^6) cells/mm^3; hence

$$MCH = \frac{15 \times 10^7}{5 \times 10^6} \qquad \text{(step 1)}$$

$$MCH = \frac{15 \times 10^{7-6}}{5} \qquad \text{(step 2)}$$

$$MCH = \frac{15 \times 10}{5} \qquad \text{(step 3)}$$

$$MCH = \frac{150}{5} \qquad \text{(step 4)}$$

$$MCH = 30 \text{ pg hemoglobin/erythrocyte} \qquad \text{(step 5)}$$

Notice step 3.

$$MCH = \frac{15 \times 10}{5} = \frac{15 \text{ (Hb in grams)} \times 10}{5 \text{ (RBC in millions)}} = \frac{15 \times 10}{5} = 30 \text{ pg}$$

Again, formula 3 is usually given because it is simple and because the numbers give the correct answer.

Mean corpuscular hemoglobin concentration

The mean* corpuscular hemoglobin concentration is the *percent* of hemoglobin in the patient's packed cell volume. Normal values range from 33% to 38%. The following is the formula for the mean corpuscular hemoglobin concentration:

$$MCHC = \frac{\text{Hb in grams} \times 100}{\text{Hct}} \qquad \text{(formula 5)}$$

The mean corpuscular hemoglobin concentration is the *percent* of hemoglobin in the packed cell volume. If the number of grams of hemoglobin in 100 ml of blood is divided by the number of milliliters of packed cells in 100 ml of blood and then this number multiplied by 100, the result would be percent of hemoglobin in the packed cell volume.

$$MCHC = \frac{\text{Grams of Hb in 100 ml blood}}{\text{Milliliters of packed cells in 100 ml blood}} \times 100 \qquad \text{(formula 6)}$$

The numerator is the number of grams of hemoglobin per 100 ml of blood (gm%).

To find the milliliters of packed cells in 100 ml blood, the denominator, take the amount of blood (100 ml) and multiply it by the percent of packed cells (in this case 50%).

$$100 \times 0.50 = 50 \text{ ml packed cells}$$

---

*Using the term *mean* in the name is not mathmatically correct. Whenever the word *average* or *mean* is used in connection with a mathematical formula, it indicates that the number of particles used to arrive at the average must be included in the denominator. In the formula for the MCHC this does not occur. The formula, in reality, finds the number of grams of hemoglobin per milliliter of packed cells and then multiplies this by 100 to arrive at a *percent*.

To work the formula, fill in the preceding information.

$$MCHC = \frac{15 \times 100}{50} \qquad \text{(step 1)}$$

$$MCHC = \frac{1500}{50} \qquad \text{(step 2)}$$

$$MCHC = 30\% \qquad \text{(step 3)}$$

Look at step 1.

$$MCHC = \frac{15 \times 100}{50} = \frac{15 \text{ (Hb in grams)} \times 100}{50 \text{ (Hct)}} = \frac{15 \times 100}{50} = 30\%$$

Examine the short formulas 1, 3, and 5 and be sure it is understood why they may be used and exactly what they represent.

Since the mean corpuscular hemoglobin concentration (MCHC) is the ratio of the mass of the mean corpuscular hemoglobin (MCH) to the mean corpuscular volume (MCV) expressed as percent, any one of these values can be calculated from the other two. The following are the formulas for these calculations:

$$MCHC = \frac{MCH}{MCV} \times 100$$

$$MCH = 0.01 \; MCHC \times MCV$$

$$MCV = \frac{MCH}{0.01 \; MCHC}$$

HEMOGLOBIN CURVE: USING CYANMETHEMOGLOBIN METHOD

The following is a basic formula that may be used to establish a hemoglobin curve:

$$\frac{\text{Concentration of standard} \times \text{Dilution factor}}{1000} = gm\%$$

The concentration of the standard is the assay on the bottle. For example, it may state 80 mg% on the front of the bottle; this is the assay or concentration.

The dilution factor is for the blood dilution made in that particular procedure. For example, if 0.02 ml blood is added to 5.0 ml diluent, the blood dilution is 0.02/5.02, or

$$\frac{0.02}{5.02} = \frac{1}{X}$$
$$0.02X = 5.02$$
$$X = 251$$
$$1/251 \text{ dilution}$$
$$\text{Dilution factor} = 251$$

As was true in an earlier chapter, the concentration of the standard for any procedure depends on the amount of blood giving the same intensity of color. The assay on the bottle (in this case 80 mg%) means that that intensity of color was produced by 80 mg% hemoglobin; that is, there are 80 mg of hemoglobin in 100 ml solution. If the test sample gives the same intensity of color, then in that test sample there are 80 mg/dl hemoglobin. But if the sample had been diluted 1/251, then whole blood would contain 251 times as much hemoglobin. Therefore, multiply the assay times the blood dilution to get the amount of hemoglobin in whole (undiluted) blood.

$$80 \times 251 = 20,080 \text{ mg/dl}$$

However, hemoglobin values are reported in gm% *(not mg%)*. Mg% may be converted to gm% by dividing by 1000.

$$\frac{80 \times 251}{1000} = 20.08 \text{ gm\%}$$

The value for this standard in *this* procedure is 20.08 gm%. This is the highest value for the standard. To set up a curve, make dilutions of the standard and calculate the corresponding values. Study the following examples:

	Amount* of diluent (ml)	Amount of standard (ml)	Value of standard (gm%)
EXAMPLE 1:			
Pure standard	0	5	20
First dilution	1	4	16
Second dilution	2	3	12
Third dilution	3	2	8
Fourth dilution	4	1	4
Pure diluent	5	0	0
EXAMPLE 2:			
Pure standard	0	8	20
First dilution	2	6	15
Second dilution	4	4	10
Third dilution	6	2	5
Pure diluent	8	0	0

*The actual amount is not important so long as the minimum quantity demanded by the instrument is available. It is the way the standard is diluted that is important. The correct value must be calculated; notice the two preceding examples.

The values for the diluted standards may be calculated two ways: (1) as a dilution problem and (2) as a ratio-proportion problem. Look at the first dilution in example 1 and consider the following two solutions:

1. As a dilution problem:

$$20 \text{ gm\%} \times \frac{4}{5} \text{ (4 ml std + 1 ml diluent = 5 ml total volume)} = 16 \text{ gm\%}$$

2. As a ratio-proportion problem: If there are 20 gm% in 5 ml, there will be X gm% in 4 ml.

$$\frac{20}{5} = \frac{X}{4}$$
$$5X = 80$$
$$X = 16 \text{ gm\%}$$

Try to determine the concentration for the first dilution in example 2.

These samples are read in the instrument, and the readings and corresponding values are plotted on the appropriate graph paper.

Practice problems

1. In a WBC wipette, blood is drawn to the 0.5 mark and diluted to the 11 mark. What is the dilution?
2. If blood is drawn to the 0.2 mark in a WBC pipette and diluted to the 11 mark, what is the dilution? What is the dilution factor?

3. In a RBC pipette, blood is drawn to the 0.8 mark and diluted to the 101 mark. What is the dilution?

4. If blood is drawn to the 1 mark in a RBC pipette and diluted to the 101 mark, what is the dilution?

5. Blood is drawn to the 0.3 mark in a WBC pipette. Ten WBC squares are counted. Give the following:
   a. Dilution factor
   b. Depth factor
   c. Area factor
   d. Volume correction factor
   e. Final factor

6. Look at Fig. 11-8. Give the following:

   Length of

   A.
   B.
   C.
   D.
   E.

   Area of

   F.
   G.
   H.
   I.

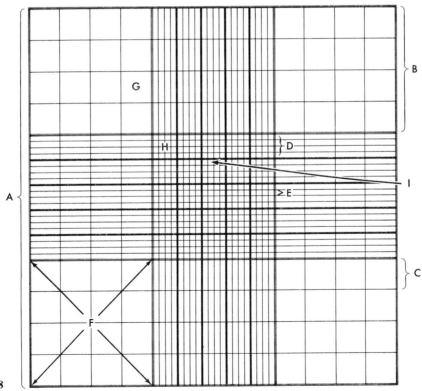

Fig. 11-8

7. In a certain platelet count procedure, one may be asked to draw the blood to the 1 mark in a RBC pipette, count all nine squares on both sides of the counting chamber, and get the average for each side. Give the following:
   a. Dilution factor
   b. Area factor
   c. Final factor

8. If 102 platelets were counted on both sides of the chamber in problem 7, what would the platelet count be?

9. A WBC count of 50,000 has been obtained. 150 NRBC/100 WBC is found on doing the differential. Give the following:
   a. Corrected WBC count
   b. NRBC/mm^3

10. RBC = 5,100,000, Hb = 15.5 gm, and Hct = 45%; give the following:
    a. MCV
    b. MCH
    c. MCHC

11. In a given hemoglobin procedure 0.05 ml blood is diluted with 6 ml diluent. The standard used for the curve is assayed at 90 mg%. What would be the highest value for this standard in this procedure? Explain exactly how a curve would be set up for this procedure using this standard. Show all work.

CHAPTER 12

Enzyme calculations

This chapter is concerned mainly with the mathematical calculations necessary to determine enzyme activity in international units and the conversion of conventional units to the newer, more consistant international units.

An enzyme reaction is a complex biochemical process in which an enzyme present in the biological sample combines with a substrate to form an enzyme-substrate complex. The complex then separates into a reaction product, or products, releasing the enzyme. The released enzyme molecule can usually repeat the reaction. Because an enzyme can enter into a reaction and remain unchanged, it is referred to as a catalyst:

$$S + E \rightleftarrows ES \rightleftarrows P + E$$

where S is the substrate; E, enzyme; P, product; and ES, enzyme-substrate complex.

Enzyme activity is usually determined either by the kinetic or the endpoint method. In the *kinetic method* the rate of the enzyme-catalyzed reaction is measured while the reaction is in progress. In the *endpoint method* a product or residual reactant is color complexed with a suitable reagent after the completion of the enzyme-catalyzed reaction. The absorbance of the complex is then measured.

KINETIC METHOD

The reaction rate is proportional to time and enzyme concentration. The concentration of the substrate must be relatively large in comparison to the quantity of enzyme present, so that the reaction rate will be independent of substrate concentration. The enzyme concentration and the time interval of the reaction will determine the quantity of substrate consumed or the amount of product formed:

$$Q = E \times t$$

where Q is the quantity of product formed; E, enzyme concentration; and t, time interval of reaction.

If the quantity of enzyme is doubled, the rate of the reaction will be doubled. The quantity of product formed in a fixed interval of time will then be doubled.

$$Q = (t) \times E$$
$$Q = 2 \times 4$$
$$Q = 8$$

If E is doubled

$$Q = 2 \times 8$$
$$Q = 16$$

Likewise, if the concentration of enzyme is kept constant and the reaction period is doubled, the amount of product formed will be doubled.

$$Q = (E) \times t$$
$$Q = 4 \times 2$$
$$Q = 8$$

If t is doubled

$$Q = 4 \times 4$$
$$Q = 16$$

As can be seen from the preceding equations, the quantity of product formed or substrate consumed is a straight line function of either enzyme concentration or time, providing the other is kept constant. If $Q = E \times t$, then $Q/t = E$, where Q/t is the rate of product formed.

Hence, the *rate* of product formation or substrate utilization may be used as a means of determining the enzyme concentration. This can be done conveniently and efficiently by spectrophotometry if one of the reactants or products is a chromogen, that is, a light absorbing substance. The change in absorbance of the reacting solution over a period of time can be measured ($\Delta A/\Delta t$). With proper concentration of initial substrate, the absorbance change (increase in product or decrease in substrate) is *directly proportional* to the activity of the enzyme. If the activity of the enzyme is doubled the rate will also be doubled. Therefore, the following is true:

$$\text{Enzyme activity} = \text{K} \frac{\Delta A}{\Delta t}$$

The constant, K, is a function of temperature, pH, sample volume, and substrate concentration.

INTERNATIONAL UNIT

As the field of enzymology progressed and new enzymes were discovered and analyzed, their activity was expressed in various units. In some cases different units were used to express the activity of the same enzyme. In 1961, the International Union of Biochemistry, through its Commission on Enzymes, recommended a standard unit known as the *international unit,* which was defined as follows: One unit (U) of any enzyme is that which will catalyze the transformation of 1 μmole of the substrate per minute under standard conditions. Concentration is to be expressed in terms of units per milliliter (U/ml) of serum, or milliunits per milliliter (mU/ml), which is the same as units per liter (U/l), whichever gives the more convenient numerical value.

$$\text{International units} = \mu\text{moles/min/ml (or liter) of serum}$$

Whereas the 1961 report of the International Union of Biochemistry recommended 25°C for the temperature of the determination, the 1964 commission suggested a change to 30°C.

The most widely used method for kinetic enzyme determinations is the *optical test* method introduced by Otto Warburg in 1936. This method is based on the fact that reduced nicotinamide adenine dinucleotide (NADH) absorbs light with an absorption maximum at 340 nm, whereas the oxidized form (NAD) shows no absorption between 300 and 400 nm. Reactions based on these compounds can involve either oxidation of NADH to NAD or the reduction of NAD to NADH. In the first case the absorbance at 340 nm decreases during the reaction; in the second case it increases.

The following explanation of the derivation or source of the basic formula for calculating international units may seem confusing at first. Read through *all* the explanation before giving up. Do *not* try to understand each sentence by itself.

The molar absorptivity of NADH at 340 nm is 6.22×10^3; that is, a solution containing 1 mole NADH/l has an absorbance of $6.22 \times 10^3 \ A$ in a cell of 1-cm path length. Therefore, a change in concentration of 1 mole/l/min would produce a change in absorbance of $6.22 \times 10^3 \ A$/min. Translation of this relationship to conditions encountered experimentally is summarized as follows:

Absorbance change per minute	Change in concentration per minute
6.22×10^3	1 mole/l
6.22×10^{-3}	1 μmole/l
6.22	1 μmole/ml
$6.22/V_t$	1 μmole in V_t ml

where V_t is the total volume of substrate and sample. Therefore, if

$$\frac{6.22}{V_t} \Delta A = 1 \ \mu\text{mole/min change in substrate}$$

then

$$1 \ \Delta A = \frac{V_t}{6.22} \ \mu\text{moles/min change in substrate}$$

If a change of ΔA/min is observed with a sample of serum volume, V_s, then

$$\Delta A/\text{min}/V_s \ \text{ml} = \Delta A/\text{min} \times \frac{V_t}{6.22} \ \mu\text{moles/min}/V_s \text{ of serum}$$

$$= \Delta A/\text{min} \times \frac{V_t}{6.22 \times V_s} \ \mu\text{moles/min/ml of serum}$$

To convert to 1 liter

$$= \Delta A/\text{min} \times \frac{V_t \times 1000}{6.22 \times V_s} \ \mu\text{moles/min/l of serum} = \text{IU/l}$$

This is the basic equation for the conversion of absorbance data to international units (IU) in procedures using NADH or NAD. This equation must be further modified to include additional factors if the following are true:
1. The activity is determined at one temperature but reported at another.
2. The molar absorptivity is affected by instrument characteristics.
   It might be helpful to think about the preceding equation in another way.

$$6.22 \ A = 1 \ \mu\text{mole/min/ml of substrate}$$

If the volume of the substrate, sample, and reagents (the total volume) is more or less than 1 ml, then it becomes necessary to divide by that amount to give the absorbance change per milliliter. Therefore

$$\frac{6.22}{V_t} A = 1 \ \mu\text{mole/min/ml}$$

where V_t is total volume. Then

$$1 \ \Delta A = \frac{V_t}{6.22} \ \mu\text{moles/min/ml}$$

or

$$\Delta A \times \frac{V_t}{6.22} = \mu\text{moles/min/ml}$$

If the change in absorbance is brought about by 1 ml of serum, then 1 ml of serum contains that number of μmoles/min/ml of serum. If other than 1 ml of serum is used in the test, it must be taken into consideration by inserting the correction factor $1/V_s$; where V_s is the volume of sample used

$$\Delta A/\text{min} \times \frac{V_t}{6.22} \times \frac{1}{V_s} = \mu\text{moles/min/ml of serum}$$

therefore

$$\frac{\Delta A \times V_t}{6.22 \times V_s} = \mu\text{moles/min/ml serum} = \text{IU/ml}$$

To convert this to μmoles/min/liter of serum, it is necessary to multiply by 1000. Finally,

$$\frac{\Delta A \times V_t \times 1000}{6.22 \times V_s} = \mu\text{moles/min/l} = \text{IU/l}$$

The preceding formula assumes a reaction time of one minute. If the reaction time is other than one minute, the factor, $1/t$, must be added to the formula.

$$\frac{\Delta A/\text{min} \times V_t}{6.22 \times V_s} \times 1000 \times \frac{1}{t} = \text{IU/l}$$

Although a wavelength setting of 340 nm is generally used to measure enzyme activity when NADH or NAD is used as substrate, 334 nm or 366 nm can be used if appropriate correction factors are applied. For example, 366 nm is recommended when a turbid serum sample or control used with a high absorbance substrate causes the initial absorbance at 340 nm to exceed the absorbance specification of the spectrophotometer. The analyst must recognize the following differences in molar absorptivity at various wavelengths.

Wavelength	Molar absorptivity
334 nm	6.0×10^3
340 nm	6.22×10^3
366 nm	3.3×10^3

The basic formula for calculation of international units is based on a molar absorptivity for NADH of 6.22×10^3 at 340 nm. If a wavelength setting of 334 nm is used, the equation must be modified by replacing 6.22 with 6.0; if 366 nm is used, 6.22 is replaced by 3.3.

CONVERSION OF CONVENTIONAL UNITS TO INTERNATIONAL UNITS
Non-NADH methods

To convert conventional units, from tests using other than NADH methods, to international units, factors for each of the parts involved in the calculations must be used. These parts of the calculations are the mass of the substrate or product, the time over which the reaction is based, and the volume of the sample solution. Normally corrections for temperature and pH are unnecessary.

Remember that 1 IU is defined as that amount of enzyme necessary to bring about the reaction of 1 μmole of substrate in one minute. These units are reported as international units per milliliter or units per liter, whichever results in the most convenient number. Other systems often use different quantities of mass, time, and volume as a base for their units. Hence, in the conversion of conventional units to international units, the mass of the substrate must be converted to micromoles, the reaction time must be converted to one minute, and the amount of the sample solution must be converted to either milliliters or liters.

EXAMPLE: How would King-Armstrong acid phosphatase units be converted to IU/l?

One KA unit is the amount of phosphatase enzyme per 100 ml of serum that will split 1 mg of phenol from phenolphosphate in 60 min.

$$1 \text{ KA unit} = 1 \text{ mg phenol}/60 \text{ min}/100 \text{ ml serum}$$
$$1 \text{ IU/l} = 1 \text{ } \mu\text{mole/min/l of serum}$$

To convert King-Armstrong units to international units, make the following calculations:
1. Convert mg to μg by multiplying by 1000.
2. Convert μg to μmoles by dividing by the molecular weight of phenol (94).
3. Convert 60 min to 1 min by dividing by 60.
4. Convert 100 ml serum to 1 liter by multiplying by 10.

This results in the following equation:

$$1 \text{ KA unit} = \frac{1000}{94} \times \frac{1}{60} \times 10 \text{ IU/l}$$

$$1 \text{ KA unit} = 1.77 \text{ IU/l}$$

NADH methods

To convert units from a test using the NADH method, but reporting in other than international units, the same basic information is sought.

EXAMPLE: Convert Karmen transaminase units to IU/l.

One Karmen transaminase unit is the amount of enzyme that will produce $\Delta 0.001$ *A* of NADH/min/ml of serum (in a total volume of 3 ml).

$$1 \text{ Karmen unit} = \Delta 0.001 \text{ } A/\text{min/ml of serum}$$
$$\text{Wanted: } \mu\text{moles/min/l}$$

$$1 \text{ Karmen unit} = \frac{0.001 \times 3}{6.22} \times 1000$$

$$1 \text{ Karmen unit} = 0.482 \text{ } \mu\text{moles/min/l} = 0.482 \text{ IU/l}$$

Notice that in either case the information desired is μmoles/min/l (or ml).

Computation of enzyme units

One of the basic formulas for calculating international units has been presented along with a method of converting some conventional units to international units.

The following presentation is a slightly rearranged, yet really more basic, computation of enzyme units (IU). Recall the information presented in Chapter 9 on molar absorptivity and the information presented in this chapter about international units. The following computations utilize the same information in a *slightly* different form. Why do the two different presentations give the same answer? Where do the differences lay?

Units of enzyme activity are computed with reference to a reaction product. The computation can be based on a *standard* by preparing a solution with an exactly known concentration of the reaction product. An aliquot of the standard solution is treated and measured together with the sample.

A standard is not required if the molar absorption coefficient, ϵ, of a reaction product is known at a given wavelength, for example, for NADH (and NADPH).

Calculation based on a standard

$$\frac{A \text{ of sample}}{A \text{ of standard}} \times 10^6 \times \text{Standard} \times \frac{1}{t} \times \frac{V_t}{V_s} = \text{IU/l}$$

when standard is concentration of the standard (moles/liter) in the assay volume; t, reaction time in minutes; V_t, total assay volume; V_s, volume of sample; IU/l, μmoles/min/l; and 10^6, factor to convert moles/l or mmoles/ml into μmoles/l.

EXAMPLE: Alkaline phosphatase.

$$p\text{-nitrophenlyphosphate} \rightleftarrows p\text{-nitrophenol} + \text{phosphate}$$

The standard is p-nitrophenol; stock solution, 1×10^{-3} moles/l; concentration in the assay mixture, 9×10^{-6}; V_t, 555 μl; V_s, 5 μl (for example, serum); t, 30 min; A of sample, 0.080; and A of standard, 0.169.

$$\frac{0.080}{0.169} \times 10^6 \times 9 \times 10^{-6} \times \frac{1}{30} \times \frac{555}{5} = 15.7 \text{ IU/l}$$

Calculation based on the molar extinction coefficient of a reaction product, with the absorbance

$$\frac{A \text{ of sample}}{\epsilon \times d} \times 10^6 \times \frac{1}{t} \times \frac{V_t}{V_s} = \text{IU/l}$$

where ϵ is molar extinction coefficient and d is diameter of the cuvette (lightpath) in centimeters. Using the preceding sample, ϵ_{400nm}, p-nitrophenol = 18.8×10^3, and $d = 1$.

$$\frac{0.080}{18.8 \times 10^3} \times 10^6 \times \frac{1}{30} \times \frac{555}{5} = 15.7 \text{ IU/l}$$

Practice problems

Convert the following to international units per liter:

1. One King-Armstrong (KA) alkaline phosphatase unit is the amount of enzyme that will split 1 mg of phenol from phenyl phosphate in 30 min at 37°C and at a pH of 9.6. It is reported per 100 ml serum. 1 KA unit/100 ml serum = 1 mg phenol/30 min/100 ml serum. 1 KA unit equals how many IU/l?
2. One Shinowara-Jones-Reinhard (SJR) alkaline phosphatase unit is the amount of enzyme that will split 1 mg phosphorus from β-glycerophosphate in 60 min at 37°C and at a pH of 9.8. It is reported per 100 ml of serum. 1 SJR unit/100 ml = 1 mg phosphorus/60 min/100 ml serum. 1 SJR unit/100 ml equals how many IU/l?
3. A de la Huerga unit for serum cholinesterase is defined as the quantity of enzyme present in 1 ml of serum that will hydrolyze 1.0 μmole of acetylcholine in 60 min, under the conditions of the assay. 1 de la Huerga unit = 1 μmole/60 min/ml. 1 de la Huerga unit equals how many IU/l?
4. In a lactic dehydrogenase procedure, 1 spectrophotometric unit is defined as the amount of enzyme that will give a $\Delta 0.001$ A change per min per ml of serum (in a total volume of 3 ml). 1 spectrophotometric unit = ΔA of 0.001/min/ml (in a total volume of 3 ml). 1 spectrophotometric unit equals how many IU/l?

CHAPTER 13

Gastric acidity

The hydrochloric acid concentration of the contents of the stomach is a value that must frequently be determined in the clinical laboratory. Two methods are currently being used in the description of the HCl concentration of this material. The older method reports the acidity in clinical units or degrees (for which the symbol "°" is used) per 100 ml of gastric contents. The newer method uses the number of milliequivalents of HCl per liter of gastric material (mEq/l).

The use of clinical units or degrees of gastric acidity is based on some physiological principles whose validity are currently being questioned. The hydrochloric acid in the gastric secretion was thought to consist of two distinct phases. According to this theory, the relative amounts of HCl in each phase are dependent on the pH of the material. If the pH is greater than 3.5, the acid is considered to be present almost exclusively as a mixture of organic salts formed from the combination of the acid with the proteins and peptones in the gastric secretion. This is called the *combined acid* and is thought to reflect the buffering capacity of the gastric proteins. Supposedly, it is only when this buffering capacity is exceeded that the HCl can exist in the second phase. In this phase the acid is in the form of dissociated ions. This is called the *free acid* and is limited to material having a pH below 3.0. The *total acid* consists of all the stomach acid, that is, the free phase plus the combined phase. The pH of the solution is determined by titration with 0.1N sodium hydroxide (NaOH). The number of clinical units or degrees of gastric acidity is equal to the number of milliliters of 0.1N NaOH required to titrate 100 ml of the gastric contents to an endpoint. Two indicators are used with this method. The endpoint of Töpfer reagent (pH 2.8 to 3.5) is used to determine the degree of free acid. The endpoint of phenolphthalein (pH 8.2 to 10.0) can be used for determining the degrees of combined acid or the degrees of total acid.

The tests for degrees of gastric acidity may be performed in one of two ways. For lack of better names, these are called the *one-dish method* and the *two-dish method*.

ONE-DISH METHOD

As the name implies, free, combined, and total acid values are found using only one dish. To begin this procedure, place an aliquot of the gastric material in an evaporating dish. Add 1 or 2 drops Töpfer reagent and titrate to the endpoint with 0.1N NaOH. Note the number of milliliters of 0.1N NaOH required to reach the endpoint. This titration will allow the calculation of the free acid. Now add 1 or 2 drops of phenolphthalein to the sample and continue to titrate. One of two procedures may be used to continue this test. If the NaOH is contained in a relatively large pipette or buret, continue to titrate from the point reached with the Töpfer reagent until the endpoint of the phenolphthalein is reached (a definite pink). This is the number of milliliters of 0.1N NaOH required for the total acid titration. To find the combined acid value, subtract the number of milliliters of NaOH required for the free acid titration from the number required for the total acid titration.

If a small pipette is used, refill it when the phenolphthalein is added to the test material, and titrate to the endpoint. This second titration will produce the value for the combined acid. Add these two titrations to get the number of milliliters of NaOH required for the total acid.

Study the procedures for the two pipette sizes. Understand that the same answer will be produced in two ways.

TWO-DISH METHOD

This method makes use of two evaporating dishes, one to titrate the free acid and the other to titrate the total acid. Place an aliquot of gastric contents into each dish. Add 1 or 2 drops Töpfer reagent to the first dish and titrate with 0.1N NaOH. The number of milliliters of NaOH required to reach the endpoint is used to calculate the degrees of free acid.

Add 1 or 2 drops of phenolphthalein to the gastric material in the second dish. Titrate with 0.1N NaOH to the endpoint and record the amount of NaOH used. This amount is used to calculate the degrees of total acid. The combined acid is found by subtracting the degrees of free acid from the degrees of total acid. Remember that the free acid produces the pH values from 1 to 3.5; the combined acid produces the pH from 3.5 to approximately 8.2; and the total acid is responsible for pH values from 1 to approximately 8.2.

With both methods, the calculation procedures are basically the same. The number of milliliters of 0.1N NaOH required to titrate 100 milliliters of gastric contents is equal to the number of degrees or clinical units of hydrochloric acid per 100 ml of gastric material. Therefore, if the amount of gastric material used and the number of milliliters of 0.1N NaOH required to reach an endpoint are known, the number of degrees can be calculated. For example, if 100 ml of gastric contents were used in the test, then the number of degrees of acidity is equal to the number of milliliters of 0.1N NaOH used in the titration. In almost all cases, however, there are less than 100 ml of gastric material available for the test. Therefore, the titrations are performed with whatever material is present, and the degrees are calculated for the data obtained.

EXAMPLE: 5 ml gastric contents are available, and the number of milliliters of 0.1N NaOH required for the *free acid* titration is 1.2 ml. What would be the number of degrees of free acidity?

Set up a ratio-proportion problem. If it took 1.2 ml NaOH to titrate 5 ml gastric contents, it would take X ml to titrate 100 ml.

$$\frac{1.2}{5} = \frac{X}{100}$$

$$5X = 120$$

$$X = 24$$

It would have taken 24 ml 0.1N NaOH for 100 ml gastric material. Hence, the free HCL equals 24° or 24 clinical units.

The answer may also be calculated using a factor. If 5 ml of gastric material were used instead of 100 ml, that is, $^5/_{100}$ or $^1/_{20}$ of the amount required, the factor to correct for this would be 20 (recall, divide by what is used and multiply by what should have been used, that is $^{100}/_5$ or 20). Hence, multiply the number of milliliters 0.1N NaOH by the factor 20.

$$1.2 \times 20 = 24° \text{ free HCl}$$

EXAMPLE: 2 ml of gastric contents were used. The Töpfer endpoint required 0.8 ml of 0.1N NaOH, and the combined acid titration required 0.5 ml NaOH. Give degrees free acid, degrees combined acid, and degrees total acid.

The factor for 2 ml of gastric material would be

$$\frac{100}{2} = 50$$

Degrees free acid $= 0.8 \times 50 = 40°$
Degrees combined acid $= \underline{0.5} \times 50 = \underline{25°}$
Degrees total acid $= \overline{1.3} \times 50 = \overline{65°}$

METHOD REPORTING RESULTS IN MILLIEQUIVALENTS PER LITER

In recent years, several studies have indicated that the preceding concept of free and combined acid is not entirely correct. It has therefore been suggested that the older terms of *free, combined,* and *total* acid be abandoned and that a newer term and concept, *titratable acidity,* be adopted.

Titratable acidity is expressed in milliequivalents of hydrochloric acid per liter of gastric material. It is determined by titration of an aliquot of gastric contents with 0.1N NaOH to pH 7.0 to 7.4 with a pH meter or colorimetrically using phenol red as the indicator (endpoint 6.8 to 8.4). The calculations used to find the milliequivalents of hydrochloric acid per liter involve the determination of the normality of the gastric material.

EXAMPLE: If 20 ml gastric contents are available for titration and titration requires 3.2 ml of 0.1N NaOH, find the titratable acidity in mEq/l.

If the normality of the gastric contents are known, then the number of mEq/l can be calculated. Therefore, set up a $V_1 \times C_1 = V_2 \times C_2$ problem.

$$V_1 \times C_1 = V_2 \times C_2$$
$$3.2 \times 0.1 = 20 \times C_2$$
$$20C_2 = 0.32$$
$$C_2 = 0.016$$

The gastric material is 0.016N. That means that there are 0.016 eq/l or 16 mEq/l (recall, eq $\times$ 1000 = mEq).

Reconsider the reporting units for the older method. The number of milliters of 0.1N NaOH required to titrate 100 ml of gastric contents is equal to the number of degrees or clinical units per *100 ml* of gastric contents. But suppose the results are requested in milliequivalents per liter instead of degrees or clinical units. It happens that the number of *degrees per 100 ml* is also the number of *milliequivalents per liter.* Numerically they are exactly the same; therefore, if one value is known so is the other. Hence, 50° total acid would also be 50 mEq/l total acid.

EXAMPLE: 5 ml gastric material are used for titration. The titration for the total acid required 1.1 ml of 0.1N NaOH.

1. Finding degrees and clinical units:

$$\frac{100}{5} = 20 \text{ (factor)}$$

$$1.1 \times 20 = 22° \text{ total acid/100 ml gastric material}$$
$$= 22 \text{ clinical units/100 ml gastric material}$$

2. Finding mEq/l:

$$V \times C = V \times C$$
$$1.1 \times 0.1 = 5 \times C$$
$$5C = 0.11$$
$$C = 0.022\text{N} = 0.022 \text{ eq/l} = 22 \text{ mEq/l}$$

Practice problems

1. Degrees are reported per how many milliliters of gastric juice?
2. Clinical units are reported per how many milliliters of gastric juice?
3. Milliequivalents per liter are reported per how many milliliters of gastric juice?
4. A one-dish titration is performed on a 5 ml sample of gastric contents. The first titration required 1.2 ml of 0.1N NaOH, and the second titration required 0.8 ml of 0.1N NaOH. Give the free, combined, and total acid concentrations in degrees and in mEq/l.
5. The total acid for a gastric sample is 60°. The free acid concentration for the same sample is 15°. What is the combined acid value?
6. A 20 ml sample of gastric juice is titrated to pH 7.4 with phenol red. The titration required 8.2 ml of 0.1N NaOH. What is the acid concentration in mEq/l?
7. 10 ml gastric contents are titrated with 0.1N NaOH. The first titration required 0.68 ml 0.1N NaOH. The total titration required 1.9 ml of 0.1N NaOH. Give the free, combined, and total acid concentrations in degrees and in mEq/l.

CHAPTER 14

Renal clearance tests

Renal clearance is the value assigned to the rate at which the kidneys remove material from the plasma or the blood. This is a quantitative expression of the rate at which a substance is excreted by the kidneys in relation to the concentration of the same substance in the plasma. For example, if plasma passing through the kidneys contains 0.1 gm of a substance per 100 ml and 0.1 gm of this substance passes into the urine each minute, then 100 ml of plasma are *cleared* of this substance per minute. Renal clearances of material are usually expressed as milliliters of plasma cleared per minute.

EXAMPLE: The blood level of creatinine is 10 mg/dl, and the quantity of creatinine that passes into the urine per minute is 6 mg. What is the clearance of creatinine?

Set up a ratio and proportion: 100 ml blood contains 10 mg; therefore, X ml would contain 6 mg.

$$\frac{100}{10} = \frac{X}{6}$$

$$10X = 600$$

$$X = 60$$

Therefore, 60 ml blood contains 6 mg creatinine; hence, 60 ml of blood are *cleared* of that amount of creatinine.

Most clearances could be figured in this manner; however, a general formula based on the preceding relationship is usually used. This formula is

$$C = \frac{U}{P} \times V$$

where C is the plasma clearance in milliliters per minute; U, concentration of the substance in the urine; P, concentration of the substance in the plasma or blood; and V, volume of urine in milliliters per minute.

The concentration of the substance in the blood and in the urine must be expressed in the same units. This formula is usually more convenient to use than the ratio-proportion setup because the concentration of the material in the blood and urine must be determined before any total amounts of the material can be obtained.

EXAMPLE: A patient of average size was found to have a creatinine concentration in the blood of 12 mg/dl and a urine concentration of 550 mg/dl. The patient produced 3 ml urine/min. Determine the renal clearance for creatinine.

$$C = \frac{U}{P} \times V$$

$$C = \frac{550}{12} \times 3$$

$$C = 137.5 \text{ ml/min}$$

This means that 137.5 ml of blood would be cleared of creatinine per minute.

The formula

$$C = \frac{U}{P} \times V$$

would apply to individuals having an average body surface. All other factors being equal, the clearance rate is roughly proportional to the size of the kidney and the body surface area of the individual. To compensate for variations in body surface area, the formula is modified thus

$$C = \frac{U}{P} \times V \times \frac{1.73 \text{ m}^2}{A}$$

The average body surface area for an adult human is 1.73 m². The value A in the formula is the body surface area of the patient. This body surface area may be obtained from a nomogram (Appendix P). It may also be calculated using the following formula:

$$\log A = (0.425 \times \log W) + (0.725 \times \log H) - 2.144$$

where A is the body surface in square meters; W, patient's weight (mass) in kilograms; and H, patient's height in centimeters.

EXAMPLE: A creatinine clearance was performed on a male patient 1.5 m tall and weighing 65 kg. His blood contained 2.5 mg/dl creatinine. The urine creatinine was 50 mg/dl and the urine volume was 300 ml/4 hr. What was the creatinine clearance for this man?

Using the formula

$$C = \frac{U}{P} \times V \times \frac{1.73}{A}$$

determine the body surface area of the patient.

$$\log A = (0.425 \times \log W) + (0.725 \times \log H) - 2.144$$
$$\log A = (0.425 \times \log 65) + (0.725 \times \log 150) - 2.144$$
$$\log A = (0.425 \times 1.812) + (0.725 \times 2.176) - 2.144$$
$$\log A = 0.770 + 1.5776 - 2.144$$
$$\log A = 0.2036$$
$$A = 1.598 \text{ or } 1.6 \text{ m}^2$$

Convert 300 ml/4 hr urine production to ml/min.

$$300 \text{ ml}/240 \text{ min} = 1.25 \text{ ml/min}$$

$$C = \frac{U}{P} \times V \times \frac{1.73}{A}$$

$$C = \frac{50}{2.5} \times 1.25 \times \frac{1.73}{1.6}$$

Do not confuse the body surface of the patient with the correction factor resulting when the body surface is divided into the average body surface. In this case the correction factor would be $1.73/1.6 = 1.08$.

$$C = \frac{50}{2.5} \times 1.25 \times 1.08 \text{ (correction factor for body surface)}$$

$$C = 20 \times 1.25 \times 1.08$$
$$C = 27 \text{ ml/min}$$

The substances for which renal clearance tests are most frequently made are urea, creatinine, and inulin. The use of each of these in such tests is beyond the scope of the book. However, when urea clearance is measured, the amount of urine produced must be considered in a slightly different light. This is due to the tendency of the kidney tubule to reabsorb some of the urea filtered by the glomeruli. The rate of this reabsorption of urea depends on the rate of the reabsorption of water. Adjustment for this is made by the use of a modified formula when a small amount of urine is produced.

The production of a urine volume of 2.0 ml/min or more is termed maximum clearance. Under maximum clearance conditions, the same formula is used for urea as is used for creatinine, that is,

$$C = \frac{U}{P} \times V \times \frac{1.73}{A}$$

If less than 2.0 ml/min of urine is produced, this is called standard clearance, and the following formula is used:

$$C = \frac{U}{P} \times \sqrt{V} \times \frac{1.73}{A}$$

The square root of the volume of urine produced is used to compensate for the reabsorption of the urea by the renal tubules.

Because there are two sets of normal values for urea clearance, one for maximum clearance and one for standard, the urea clearance is often reported as *percent of normal*. This means the percent that the test values are of the normal range. The normal values for the maximum and standard clearances are as follows:

	Mean (ml/min)	Range (ml/min)	Range (% of normal)
Maximum	75	64 to 99	75 to 125
Standard	54	41 to 68	75 to 125

Note that the normal *range in percent of normal* is the same for both the maximum and standard clearance. To convert the clearance in milliliters per minute to percent of normal, it is necessary to expand the formulas as follows:

$$\text{Maximum } C\% \text{ of normal} = \frac{U}{P} \times V \times \frac{1.73}{A} \times \frac{100}{75}$$

$$\text{Standard } C\% \text{ of normal} = \frac{U}{P} \times \sqrt{V} \times \frac{1.73}{A} \times \frac{100}{54}$$

The numbers 75 and 54 represent the normal mean values for maximum and standard clearances, respectively.

Practice problems

1. A man weighs 220 lb and is 5 ft 10 in tall; give the following:
   a. His body surface (two ways: nomogram and formula)
   b. The factor for correcting for his body surface
2. Give the creatinine clearance for the following information: plasma creatinine is 2.0 mg/dl, urine creatinine is 50 mg/dl, and urine volume is 400 ml/4 hr.
3. A urea clearance is performed on a male patient. The plasma urea is 20 mg/dl, the urine urea is 500 mg/dl, and the urine volume is 300 ml/2 hr. Report as milliliters of plasma cleared per minute and as percent of normal.
4. The following information is available for a urea clearance test: serum urea 30 mg/dl and urine urea 5400 mg for a 24-hr specimen that had a volume of 1800 ml. The patient is 5 ft 6 in tall and weights 130 lb. Report the following:
   a. Patient's body surface
   b. Body surface correction factor
   c. Urea clearance in milliliter per minute uncorrected for body surface
   d. Urea clearance in milliliter per minute corrected for body surface
   e. Urea clearance in percent of normal corrected for body surface
   f. Urea clearance in percent of normal uncorrected for body surface

CHAPTER 15

Quality control

The control of the quality of analytical work should be an integral part of the standard operating procedure of every laboratory. This part of the laboratory activities can be divided into three phases: (1) the establishment of accurate standards with which to compare production work, (2) the evaluation of the comparison of the work with the standards, and (3) the implementation of corrective measures to improve the quality of the laboratory work. Most of the first and last of these phases is beyond the scope of this book. The second phase is discussed in some detail in this chapter.

In the establishment of comparison standards, several factors should be considered. The standards of similar laboratories, commercial suppliers, and the recommendations of the associations, boards, congresses, and other cooperative groups are usually the most convenient sources of reliable standards. A reference standard should reflect the phenomena, for which the production test is being used, to the highest degree of accuracy and precision possible. An individual laboratory may desire to develop a reference standard. This is quite feasible provided the personnel fully understand the phenomenon being evaluated and the theory and application of the test procedures.

The implementation of needed measures is the most important and often the most difficult phase of a quality control program. The most elaborate and complete evaluation of the work done by a laboratory is for naught unless some effective use is made of the information obtained.

The comparison of test results with standard values and the evaluation of these comparisons usually involve the science of statistics. Statistics includes the mathematics involved with the estimation of the significance of deviations of test values from some theoretically correct value. Statistical methods must be used in combination with good logic and common sense. Quality control programs often fail to be beneficial when the laboratory personnel try to make statistics do their thinking.

Statistics is often the basis of accidental or designed errors. We actively condemn the purposeful use of statistics to create untrue implications or to support known lies. Statistics should be used as a tool to estimate a true situation!

Quality control programs should assist in the increase of the accuracy and precision of the laboratory results. The terms accuracy and precision are often erroneously used to mean, or at least imply, the same thing. They both deal with quality, but each deals with a different property of quality.

Accuracy is used to describe the closeness of a test value to the actual value. *Precision* is used in two ways. In statistical usage it usually refers to the reproducibility of a test value, in which case it means the consistency of a series of test results. The term *reproducibility* is also often used in this manner. However, at times precision is used to denote the size of the increments used in the measure. For example, an object having a mass of exactly 1.787 kg is weighed in several ways. If it is weighed on a balance that will only weigh to the nearest kilogram and is shown to have a mass of between 1 and 2 kg, this would be an accurate measurement of its mass. However, this would be a very low degree of precision. Another weighing of the object on another balance showed the mass to be 1.27489 kg. This value would be very precise but not accurate. Next, the mass of the object was measured by five people using five different instruments. The values obtained were 1.7870, 1.787, 1.8, 1.78700, and 1.78 kg. This series of measurements would all be accurate to different numbers of significant figures. The level of precision (reproducibility) of the series would also be high, and the fourth measurement would be extremely precise in itself.

A very definite possibility of measuring devices is that they can have precision and not accuracy. In words much used, "One is often precisely wrong. One may also be approximately accurate." The degree of accuracy or precision is relative to the situation. If one measures a distance of 5 km to the nearest meter, this would probably be considered to be a high level of precision. However, if the width of a laboratory bench were measured to the nearest meter, this would be a very low degree of precision. The degree of precision necessary would depend on the situation in which the measurements are made. The term *reliability* is frequently used to describe the degree of accuracy and precision of a procedure.

In general, the evaluation of precision is easier than the evaluation of accuracy. In determining the precision of work, one needs only to calculate the *consistency* of the measurements or note the number of significant figures in the values. The degree of accuracy however, must be determined by comparing the values obtained in the laboratory work with values known to be correct. The correct values are usually obtained from standardized test materials subjected to ideal test procedures and conditions.

STATISTICAL TERMINOLOGY

Often the formulas and terminology found in statistics overwhelm the beginning student. This need not be the case if some effort is made to learn a basic language of statistics before attempting to analyze data.

Observations and variables

Observations are the recognized characteristics of something. These observations can either be qualitative or quantitative. *Qualitative observations* are descriptions of such properties as color, texture, turbidity, and odor. These are nonnumerical in value. *Quantitative observations* are descriptions that utilize numerical values. The size of an object, the concentration of a solution, and the length of time required for some event are examples of quantitative observations. Observations that are not constant are called *variables*, and variables are the raw materials for statistical methods. Only quantitative variables can be treated by these methods. Some qualitative observations can be converted to quantitative values. For example, the wavelength of light reflected determines the color of a compound. Statistics can be used with a series of wavelengths, but they cannot be used with colors.

Quantitative variables may be continuous or discrete. *Continuous variables* are those for which any value within a particular range is possible. Examples of continuous variables include the diameter of red blood cells, the concentration of a solute in a solution, and the amount of uric acid excreted in one day. Continuous variables are limited only by the precision of the measurement. *Discrete variables* are those that can vary only in minimum increments. The number of tests completed in one day, the number of basophils in a differential blood count, and the number of heartbeats per minute are all examples of discrete variables. A series of related observations is usually referred to as *data* (singular, datum).

Populations and samples

All possible values for a particular characteristic constitute a *population*. All these values do not have to be different nor does their number have to be finite. Some populations are essentially infinite, such as the differential blood counts done in the past, present, and future. Some populations are relatively small, for example, the results of tests conducted by one laboratory during one particular month. A population can be anything it is defined to be.

A *sample* is any part of a population. Usually samples are small parts of large populations and are used to make inferences of populations. For this reason samples should be chosen carefully so that they are representative of the population. This is most important if the calculations of the observations in a sample are to accurately reflect the properties of the population. For a sample to be representative of a population it has to be selected using procedures that ensure randomness. A *random sample* is one chosen so that there is no preference given to any part of the population. There has been a great deal of experimentation showing that human beings cannot select a truly random sample without the use of some nonliving process. There are many such processes that may be used to generate a random sample. The drawing of a card from a shuffled deck, the roll of dice, or the toss of a balanced coin are all means of producing a random set of numbers. The statistician usually uses either a table of random numbers or a computer to produce the order of selection used to draw a random sample.

Parameters and statistics

Calculations from data are either parameters or statistics depending on the body of data used. If some calculation is made from an entire population, the results will be only one possible value. Such values are *parameters*. *Statistics* are calculated from samples of populations. Because different samples from the same populations can vary, statistics vary. Much of the work of the statistician involves the estimation of the extent of the variation of statistics.

CALCULATED STATISTICAL VALUES

Most statistical calculations can be placed in one of two groups: measures of central tendency and measures of dispersion.

Measurements of central tendency

The most common measures of central tendency are the mean, the median, and the mode. The *mean* is the value usually referred to as the arithmetic average. This value is calculated by dividing the sum of all individual values by the number of values. When a mean is calculated from all values of a population, it is a parameter and is usually assigned the symbol "μ." When the mean is calculated from a sample of a population, it is a statistic and is represented by the symbol "$\overline{X}$" (called X-bar)

$$\mu = \frac{\Sigma X}{N} \qquad\qquad X = \frac{\Sigma X}{n}$$

where μ is the population mean; Σ, sum of; X, individual variables; N, number of values in the population; $\overline{X}$, sample mean; and n, number of variables in the sample.

The mean is the most used measure of central tendency. The value μ is a precise value for a population, whereas $\overline{X}$ is an estimate of μ based on a *sample* of that population.

The *median* is another measure of central tendency. This is the middle value of a body of data. If all the variables in the data are ranked in order of increasing magnitude, the median is that variable falling halfway between the highest and the lowest in position. In the case of a series containing an odd number of variables, the median will be the variable in the middle of the array. If the series contains an even number of observations, the median is the mean of the two middle values.

The *mode* is the most frequently occurring variable in a mass of data. This value may be any value within the body of data.

EXAMPLE: Consider the following values for the number of eosinophils in seven differential blood counts: 3,8,5,1,3,11, and 4. These counts would be a sample of a larger population unless otherwise defined. Hence all values calculated from this body of data would be statistics.

The *mean* of these values would be the sum of the values ($\Sigma X = 35$) divided by the total number of values ($n = 7$).

$$\overline{X} = \frac{\Sigma X}{n}$$

$$\overline{X} = \frac{35}{7}$$

$$\overline{X} = 5$$

The *median* would equal the middle value. To find the median, first rank the values according to magnitude: 1,3,3,4,5,8,11. There are seven values in this array. The median would be the middle value in the array. In an array of seven variables, the fourth variable from either end would be median. In this case the median is the variable 4.

median
↓
1,3,3,④,5,8,11

The *mode* is the most frequently occurring value. In this array that value is 3.

mode
1,3̑,3,4,5,8,11

Measures of dispersion

Measures of dispersion are calculated values that indicate the extent of variation of the observations. The most common measures of dispersion include the range, the variance, and the standard deviation. The *range* is the simplest measure of dispersion. This also gives the least information about the data. The range is the difference between the highest and lowest values in the sample or population. This is calculated by subtracting the lowest value from the highest.

EXAMPLE: Using the data from the sample of blood counts, calculate the range of the eosinophils in the sample. Remember that the observations are 3,8,5,1,3,11, and 4.

The lowest value is 1, and the highest value is 11; hence, $11 - 1 = 10$. The range of this sample is 10.

Variance and standard deviation are the two most commonly used measures of dispersion. The *standard deviation* is the square root of the variance. Hence, if the variance is known, the standard deviation can be easily calculated and vice versa. Both of these measures characterize the dispersion of the variables about the mean. The classic formula for the *variance* of a population sample is as follows:

$$s^2 = \frac{\Sigma (X - \overline{X})^2}{n - 1}$$

where s^2 is the variance of a sample; Σ, sum of; X, variables; $\overline{X}$, mean; and n, number of variables in the sample. Consider the preceding example. The variables of the number of eosinophils from differential blood counts are 3,8,5,1,3,11, and 4. The mean of these values is 5. To calculate the variance of the data, first calculate $X - \overline{X}$ for each variable.

X	$\overline{X}$	$X - \overline{X}$	$(X - \overline{X})^2$
3	5	-2	4
8	5	$+3$	9
5	5	0	0
1	5	-4	16
3	5	-2	4
11	5	$+6$	36
4	5	-1	1
		0	$70 = \Sigma(X - \overline{X})^2$

Note that the algebraic sum of $X - \overline{X}$ equals zero. This should be the case if the calculations are done correctly. This may vary slightly from zero if the values are rounded off. Also note that all $(X - \overline{X})^2$ values are positive, as a negative number times a negative number will yield a positive number.

Next divide $\Sigma(X - \overline{X})^2$ by the number of observations less one. One less than the number of observations is called the *degrees of freedom.*

The degrees of freedom is the number of variables in a sample or population that can be any value and still give the same result. In general, one degree of freedom is lost for every group of variables. In this case, all the variables are considered to be in one group. All the values but one could vary and still produce the same statistic. One variable must be one particular value to produce that particular statistic. Hence all variables but one have freedom. The full implication of this concept requires a study of statistics beyond the scope of this book.

The calculation

$$\frac{\Sigma(X - \overline{X})^2}{n - 1}$$

equals the variance of the data.

$$s^2 = \frac{70}{6} = 11.67$$

The standard deviation is the square root of the variance; hence, the standard deviation of the preceding data is calculated as follows:

$$s = \sqrt{s^2} = \sqrt{\frac{\Sigma(X - \overline{X})^2}{n - 1}}$$

$$s = \sqrt{11.67}$$
$$s = 3.42$$

where s is the standard deviation.

Another formula that is frequently used to calculate the variance and standard deviation is as follows:

$$s^2 = \frac{\Sigma X^2 - \frac{(\Sigma X)^2}{n}}{n - 1}$$

or

$$s = \sqrt{\frac{\Sigma X^2 - \frac{(\Sigma X)^2}{n}}{n - 1}}$$

This formula is much easier to use with most mechanical and electronic calculators. For this reason it is often referred to as the machine formula.

EXAMPLE: Consider the data used previously for the differential blood count: 3,8,5,1,3,11, and 4. Calculate the variance and standard deviation using the machine formula.

X	X^2
3	9
8	64
5	25
1	1
3	9
11	121
4	16
$\Sigma X = 35$	$\Sigma X^2 = 245$
$(\Sigma X)^2 = 1225$	

$$s^2 = \frac{\Sigma X^2 - \frac{(\Sigma X)^2}{n}}{n - 1}$$

$$s^2 = \frac{245 - \frac{(35)^2}{7}}{6}$$

$$s^2 = \frac{245 - \frac{1225}{7}}{6}$$

$$s^2 = \frac{245 - 175}{6}$$

$$s^2 = \frac{70}{6}$$

$$s^2 = 11.67$$

$$s = \sqrt{s^2}$$
$$s = \sqrt{11.67}$$
$$s = 3.42$$

The statistics or parameters, variance and standard deviation, are measures of the dispersion of a set of data around the mean. This gives an estimate of the degree of uniformity of the data. All large standard deviations in relation to the mean would indicate that the data is not very uniform. A lower standard deviation means that the data is more uniform.

Coefficient of variation

These statistics, variance and standard deviation, vary with the data considered, so it is not accurate to compare the standard deviations of two samples without also considering the mean. The *coefficient of variation* is used to make such a comparison.

This is equal to the standard deviation divided by the mean.

$$CV = \frac{s}{\overline{X}}$$

The coefficient of variation of the preceding example is calculated as follows:

$$CV = \frac{3.42}{5}$$

$$CV = 0.68$$

This value is frequently given as a percentage.

$$\%CV = \frac{s}{\overline{X}} \times 100$$

$$\%CV = \frac{3.42}{5} \times 100$$

$$CV = 68\%$$

The coefficient of variation can be used in many ways. It is useful in the comparison of the dispersion of two similar sets of data. It can be useful in comparing one day's work with a similar day or test results in one laboratory with the same type of results from another laboratory.

It is not wise to use the coefficient of variation to compare situations having several varying conditions. A coefficient of variation of 68% may be considered good for one body of data but very poor for another. As with all statistics and parameters, this should be used with care and common sense.

NORMAL DISTRIBUTION

One common way of organizing the values of the observations of a population or sample is to construct a frequency distribution from the values of the variables. A *frequency distribution* represents a comparison of the magnitude of the variables with how frequently each particular value occurs. The usual method used to present a frequency distribution is a graph. The possible values in the population are usually arranged in increasing magnitude along the horizonal axis, whereas the number of times a particular value (that is, its frequency) occurs in the population or sample is arranged along the vertical axis. The frequency of each value is plotted on the graph. The pattern of the resulting curve indicates how the values are distributed throughout the range.

Many populations form a particular kind of frequency distribution, commonly called a *normal distribution,* or Gaussian distribution. This is usually presented as a curve on a graph as described previously. Fig. 15-1 shows this curve. The curve of a normal distribution shows the frequency of values increasing until the mean is reached and then decreasing with the same slope. The curve of the normal distribution is often referred to as a bell-shaped curve. This relationship applies to a theoretical population distributed completely at random. In such a theoretical population, the mean, median, and mode will be the same.

The normal distribution is useful in statistical calculations because of the large number of populations that either form this type of frequency distribution or approach it. Also, a completely random sample drawn from such a population will have a frequency distribution very close to a normal distribution.

If a particular sample does not form a normal distribution and the population is

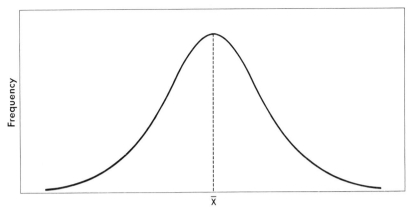

Fig. 15-1

assumed to have a normal distribution, there is a probability that the sample is not random and that the observations result from conditions different from the population from which it was thought to have been drawn.

In a normal distribution, a constant relationship exists between the shape of the distribution curve and the standard deviation of the data. This is true because both are functions of the dispersion of the data around the mean. A detailed discussion of this relationship is necessary to understand the basis of its use in quality control systems.

The curve of the normal distribution can be used to estimate the probability of a particular value occurring in a random sample. Stated very simply, probability is the chance of some event occurring. In this situation the probability is the chance of some particular value occurring in a sample. The probability of a particular value being chosen in a sample varies from 0 to 1. If a value could never occur in a sample, its probability would be zero. If a value were chosen every time in the selection of a sample, its probability would be 1. If a value occurred some of the time but not every time, its probability would be between zero and 1. This, of course, would be a fraction. Probability may be expressed in percentage. The probability values would then range from 0% to 100%. Percentage is usually more easily understood, so this will be the way in which probability is discussed here.

The curve of the frequency distribution of a population will include all the observations of the population. The area of the graph between the curve and the horizontal axis is analogous to the probability of some observation having a value between and including the lowest and the highest value in the population; this probability is 100%.

The probability of a particular observation having a value between any two points on the horizontal axis will equal the proportion of the area under the curve between two vertical lines drawn from the curve to the horizontal axis at these points.

This same general relationship is true for the frequency distribution of a random sample drawn from a population. There is one difference however. The probability of a value falling within the range of a sample will theoretically always be a little less than 100%. This will not significantly affect the considerations here, but it needs to be recognized if a more extensive study of statistics is undertaken.

In a normal distribution there is a constant relationship between the standard deviation and the probability of values occurring in a population or sample.

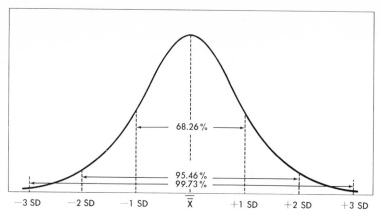

Fig. 15-2

The mean of a normally distributed body of data will be equal to the most frequently occurring value; hence, the mean will correspond to the highest point on the curve of a normal distribution.

The probability of some observation having a value between the mean and one standard deviation (1s) greater than the mean is 34.13%. This is a constant value owing to the method of calculation of the standard deviation and the construction of the normal distribution curve. As the curve is symmetrical, the same probability exists for a value between 1s less than the mean and the mean value. Hence, the probability of some value from a population or sample being within one standard deviation on either side of the mean ($\pm$1s) is 68.26% (2 $\times$ 34.13).

Study Fig. 15-2. Note that 68.26% of the area under the curve is between one standard deviation less than the mean ($-$1s) and one standard deviation greater than the mean ($+$1s). The probability of an observation having a value within $\pm$2s of the mean is 95.46%, whereas the probability of a value being within $\pm$3s of the mean is 99.73%.

This relationship between the frequency distribution curve and the standard deviation applies only to normal distributions. Not all populations will form a normal distribution. The reason for this can be found in more complete references on statistics. Be careful when using the procedures involving the standard deviations and the normal curve.

$\overline{X}$ OR LEVEY-JENNINGS CHART

The most common system of quality control in the medical laboratory involves the use of the X or Levey-Jennings chart. In general this system uses the mean and standard deviation of a series of standard tests conducted during some previous time period. The X chart is an extension of points along the horizontal axis of the graph of the normal distribution. The graph is usually turned on its side for convenience so that the horizontal axis becomes the vertical axis in this manner of presentation. Study Fig. 15-3.

The major lines of the chart are placed at the points on the axis corresponding to the mean and $\pm$1s and $\pm$2s from the mean. The probability of a standard substance producing a test value with $\pm$1s of the mean is about 68.3%. The probability of the test results of a standard being within $\pm$2s is about 95.5%. This means that every test result of the standard solution has a 68.3% chance of being within $\pm$1s of the mean established for this particular test. The chance of being within $\pm$2s of the established

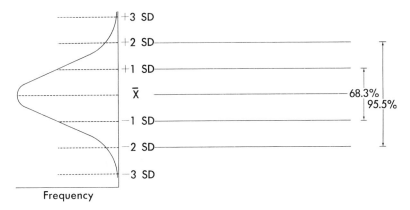

Fig. 15-3

mean is about 95.5%. This also means that each test result has a 31.7% chance of varying more than $\pm 1s$ from the mean or a 4.5% chance of varying more than $\pm 2s$ from the mean owing to random error alone. Therefore one would expect about 1 in 22 test values to vary more than $\pm 2s$ from the established mean even if the test conditions are acceptable.

The mean and standard deviations used on an $\overline{X}$ chart are determined from a series of tests on standard solutions done by the laboratory. The standard solutions are often called controls. In most situations at least one test is made per day using the control. The mean and standard deviations are calculated from the test results of the controls over a given period of time. There should be at least 20 and preferably 30 test results used in the preparation of a chart.

The mean and standard deviations calculated from the test results of the laboratory are the values that should be used for the $\overline{X}$ and s values of that laboratory.

The most common source of controls such as standard serum is from commercial suppliers. These companies establish the mean and acceptable range of the standard using results from several reference laboratories. These reference laboratories have the most accurate and precise equipment, supplies, and personnel available. These values are to be used as a guide in a quality control program of a working laboratory. They are not the values to be used on the charts of the laboratory. The results of the daily tests of the control solution within the particular laboratory are the ones to be used in the establishment of the values on the chart. The mean of the laboratory tests should be within the acceptable range provided by the suppliers, however.

The procedure used to obtain the results on the control solutions should be as nearly like the procedure used with the patient samples as possible. If possible, the analyst conducting the test should not know which sample is the control. The standard tests should be conducted at random within the normal routine of the laboratory. If more than one person conducts a particular type of test, each person involved should do some of the tests on the controls during each time period. Every standard test result should be recorded on the quality control charts. This includes tests that may have been repeated for one reason or another.

The preceding considerations are necessary if a quality control program is to accurately reflect the work production of the laboratory.

A quality control program will aid in the evaluation of the conditions under which the standard tests are conducted. If the conditions of the general laboratory work are different from the conditions of the standard tests, the quality control program is not evaluating the work of the laboratory—it is evaluating the conditions used to run the controls! This situation occurs much too frequently. Many quality control programs are conducted to satisify some regulatory or public relations requisite and not to determine the quality of the work done in the laboratory. This is very short sighted. It can only result in a false impression of the laboratory work and probably result in patient test results of lower reliability than should be tolerated.

A different $\overline{X}$ chart is set up for each procedure included in the quality control program. The magnitude of the mean and standard deviations is established using the results of the tests on the standard solutions as described earlier in this chapter.

When the mean and standard deviations are calculated, the major lines of the $\overline{X}$ chart can be established.

The results of future tests on the standards are then plotted on the chart. The pattern formed by these points can be easily studied to determine if the particular test procedure is *in control* or *out of control*. The terms, *in control* and *out of control,* are used to describe the acceptability of the reliability of the test procedures. A test under technical control at the bench level is said to be in control and has enough accuracy and precision to be used for patient testing. A test is out of control when the error associated with the procedure is too great to produce results of sufficient reliability to be used in patient diagnosis.

Since the pattern of the control test results is used to determine if a test procedure is in or out of control, this requires careful interpretation.

The limits of variation normally considered allowable for the standard test results have been established as $\pm 2s$ from the mean. If a test procedure is operating correctly, 95.5% of the control values will fall within this range. This also means that 4.5% of the values can fall outside this range due to acceptable error alone. Any interpretation of an $\overline{X}$ chart should be made using a series of test values. One value should never be used in any determination of the reliability of a test. Each value should be used in context with the other values in the series. In general, if a series of control results forms a random pattern between $+2s$ and $-2s$ on the $\overline{X}$ chart with only an occasional value falling outside this range, it is assumed that all technical phases of the test procedure are equal for all samples and that there is a high degree of probability that the patient values are correct and can be relied on in the formation of a diagnosis. However, this does not preclude the possibility that a particular patient sample may be tested so as to produce an erroneous result. As with all phases of laboratory technique, careful work and good logic are very necessary.

An occasional value falling outside the $\pm 2s$ limit may or may not be significant. One common practice in this situation is to repeat the control test. If the repeat result is within the $\pm 2s$ limit, it can be assumed that the wide ranging value was due to chance alone and not to some problem with the procedure. If the second test produces a value outside the accepted limits, the test procedure should be examined to determine the cause of the aberrant results. Patient values should not be reported until the problem is found and corrected. In either case, all results of the tests of the control should be plotted on the chart.

Another generalization in the interpretation of the control values is that if six successive plots fall on the mean line or on one side of the mean line, the procedure is considered out of control. This condition is known as a shift. The mean of these tests has shifted from the established mean. The procedure should be examined to identify the problem and correct it. The placement of six plots on one side of the mean has been established as the most practical for the majority of clinical laboratories.

Another common situation seen on the $\overline{X}$ chart is that referred to as a trend. A trend is indicated by six successive plots being distributed in one general direction on the chart. This is another condition indicating that the test is out of control. Again, the test procedure should be examined and adjusted as with a shift.

Study the following examples, which include some of the most common types of situations found in the quality control programs of the clinical laboratory.

Figure 15-4 shows an $\overline{X}$ chart for the BUN procedure of a particular laboratory for the month of April. The mean and standard deviations used for this chart were calculated from the control values for the month of March. Fig. 15-5 shows these values with the calculations. This type of work sheet is provided by several companies. Many laboratories make their own. It helps to organize the calculations, and this type of chart may prove helpful for some people.

The chart in Fig. 15-4 shows that the test procedure is in control. The results of the control tests are distributed along each side of the mean in a random manner. Note the plot ⊡ at day 24. This value was outside the $\pm 2s$ limit of the chart. The control test was repeated, and the plot ⊙ resulted. The second value fell within the acceptable limits, so the outlying value is considered to be due to random error and is acceptable. All values on this chart, including the outlier, should be used to calculate the mean and standard deviation for the chart to be used during the next test period.

The values of the April chart were used to calculate the mean and standard deviation for the May chart shown in Fig. 15-6.

The May chart shows a common situation in this type of quality control program. The control test for day seven gave a result outside the $\pm 2s$ limit (plot △). The test was repeated and gave the plot ⊡. The second value for day seven was also outside the acceptable limits, indicating an out-of-control situation. The reagents used in the procedure were examined and were found to be contaminated. These were replaced and a third control test was conducted. The results of this test gave plot ⊙, and the test was back in control.

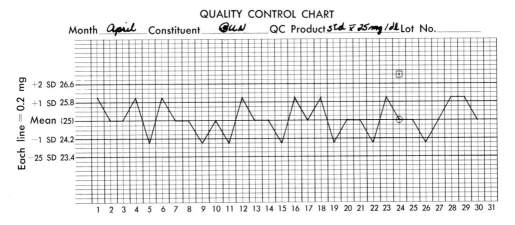

Fig. 15-4

DATE	ANALYST	DETERMINATION	TRUE VALUE	AVERAGE
march		*BUN*	*25 mg/dl*	

Procedure for Calculating Average and Standard Deviation

1. Record each observation in column "x".

2. Add the values in column "x" and divide by the number of observations.

3. Calculate and record the differences between the average value and each individual observation in column "d".

4. Square each individual difference and record in column "d²".

5. Add the squared differences.

6. Calculate S.D. using formula.

Calculations

Average $\bar{x} = \dfrac{\Sigma x}{n} = \dfrac{775}{31} = 25$

where Σ = sum of

x = each individual observation

n = total number of observation $= 31$

Standard Deviation $\sigma = \sqrt{\dfrac{\Sigma (\bar{x}-x)^2}{n-1}} = \dfrac{20}{30} = .8165$

σ = standard deviation =

Σ = sum of

x = each individual observation

x = average value $= 25$

© COPYRIGHT 1964 GENERAL DIAGNOSTICS

#	x	d	d²
1.	25	0	
2.	25	0	
3.	24	1	1
4.	25	0	
5.	26	1	1
6.	27.25	2,0	4
7.	26	1	1
8.	25	0	
9.	25	0	
10.	24	1	1
11.	24	1	1
12.	26	1	11
13.	25	0	
14.	24	1	1
15.	25	0	
16.	25	0	
17.	24	1	1
18.	25	0	
19.	26	1	1
20.	25	0	
21.	26	1	1
22.	26	1	1
23.	25	0	
24.	24	1	1
25.	25	0	
26.	24	1	1
27.	26	1	1
28.	25	0	
29.	24	1	1
30.	24	1	1
31.			
			20

Fig. 15-5. Standard deviation work sheet.

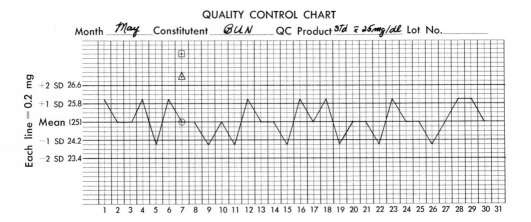

QUALITY CONTROL CHART

Month *May* Constitutent *BUN* QC Product *Std x̄ 25mg/dl* Lot No. _____

Each line = 0.2 mg

+2 SD 26.6
+1 SD 25.8
Mean (25)
−1 SD 24.2
−2 SD 23.4

1 2 3 4 5 6 7 8 9 10 11 12 13 14 15 16 17 18 19 20 21 22 23 24 25 26 27 28 29 30 31

Fig. 15-6

The values of the May test are used to calculate the mean and standard deviation used on the June chart. This raises the question as to whether or not to use the control values that detected an out-of-control situation. On this particular chart, this would include the first two control values for day seven. We know of no authorities who discuss this problem. However, since the $\overline{X}$ chart is based on a normal distribution, it is recommended that only those values that are part of a randomly distributed set of control values should be used in the determination of the mean and standard deviations to be used on a quality control chart. Since the results of the first two control tests for day seven were not part of the random distribution of the values for May, they should not be used in the calculation of the statistics for the June chart. They should, however, *appear* on the May chart.

An example of a $\overline{X}$ chart showing a shift is presented in Fig. 15-7. The shift is the control values from day 17 through day 22. The sixth consecutive value above the mean (plot ⊙) confirmed an out-of-control situation. The procedure was examined, and the problem was corrected. The plot of day 23 showed the procedure to be back in control.

Fig. 15-8 shows a chart demonstrating a trend. The values from day 17 through

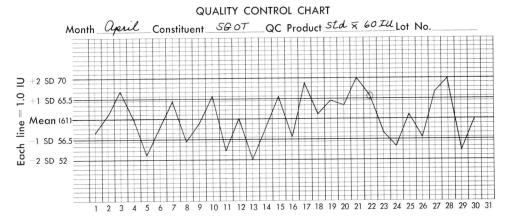

Fig. 15-7

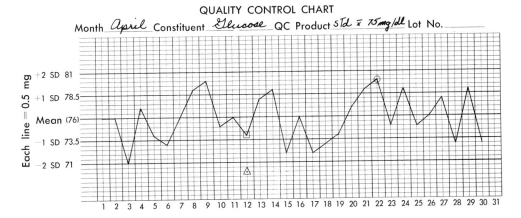

Fig. 15-8

22 shows a series of increasing values. The procedure for glucose determination was examined and the problem corrected, as seen by the position of the plot for day 23.

When using the values on both of these charts to calculate the statistics for the next chart, one should not use the values that indicated the shift and the trend. These values were subject to conditions not common to the values indicating that the procedure was in control. Many technologists use these values as a matter of course. This practice will result in a change of the mean and the standard deviations of the next month's chart, and the change would be due to values that indicated an out-of-control condition. These values are bias and are not part of a random sample.

In Fig. 15-8 a control value fell outside the $\pm 2s$ limit at day 12 (plot △). Another control test was made and resulted in plot ⊡. The first plot was due to random error and did not indicate an out-of-control situation.

The foregoing discussion of statistics is useful for the day-to-day quality control programs of the clinical laboratory. It is a limited discussion of the use of statistics. The science of statistics includes much more than what is discussed here. This area of mathematics is so extensive that even a beginning study requires much more detail material than would be appropriate in this book. Many good books exist for most any program of study of statistics. If more information is desired in this area, the reader should refer to more complete statistical works.

Alphabet table

Greek letter	Greek name	English equivalent
A α	Alpha	(ä)
B β	Beta	(b)
Γ γ	Gamma	(g)
Δ δ	Delta	(d)
E ε	Epsilon	(e)
Z ζ	Zeta	(z)
H η	Eta	(ā)
Θ θ	Theta	(th)
I ι	Iota	(ē)
K κ	Kappa	(k)
Λ λ	Lambda	(l)
M μ	Mu	(m)
N ν	Nu	(n)
Ξ ξ	Xi	(ks)
O o	Omicron	(ǫ)
Π π	Pi	(p)
P ρ	Rho	(r)
Σ σ ς	Sigma	(s) 6
T τ	Tau	(t)
Υ υ	Upsilon	(ü, ōō)
Φ φ	Phi	(f)
X χ	Chi	(H)
Ψ ψ	Psi	(ps)
Ω ω	Omega	(ō)

Modified from Weast, R. C., editor: Handbook of chemistry and physics, ed. 46, Cleveland, Ohio, 1965, CRC Press, Inc., p. F-139.

Cardinal numbers: Arabic and Roman

Name	Arabic symbol	Roman symbol
Naught, zero, or cipher	0	
One	1	I
Two	2	II
Three	3	III
Four	4	IV
Five	5	V
Six	6	VI
Seven	7	VII
Eight	8	VIII
Nine	9	IX
Ten	10	X
Eleven	11	XI
Twelve	12	XII
Thirteen	13	XIII
Fourteen	14	XIV
Fifteen	15	XV
Sixteen	16	XVI
Seventeen	17	XVII
Eighteen	18	XVIII
Nineteen	19	XIX
Twenty	20	XX
Twenty-one	21	XXI
Twenty-two	22	XXII
Thenty-three	23	XXIII
Twenty-four	24	XXIV
Twenty-five	25	XXV
Twenty-six	26	XXVI
Twenty-seven	27	XXVII
Twenty-eight	28	XXVIII
Twenty-nine	29	XXIX
Thirty	30	XXX
Thirty-one	31	XXXI
Forty	40	XL
Forty-one	41	XLI
Fifty	50	L
Sixty	60	LX
Seventy	70	LXX
Eighty	80	LXXX
Ninety	90	XC
One hundred	100	C
One hundred and one or one hundred one	101	CI
Two hundred	200	CC
Three hundred	300	CCC
Four hundred	400	CD
Five hundred	500	D
Six hundred	600	DC
Seven hundred	700	DCC
Eight hundred	800	DCCC

Name	Arabic symbol	Roman symbol
Nine hundred	900	CM
One thousand or ten hundred	1000	M
Two thousand	2000	MM
Five thousand	5000	$\overline{V}$
Ten thousand	10,000	$\overline{X}$
One hundred thousand	100,000	$\overline{C}$
One million	1,000,000	$\overline{M}$

Ordinal numbers

Name	Symbol
First	1st
Second	2d or 2nd
Third	3d or 3rd
Fourth	4th
Fifth	5th
Sixth	6th
Seventh	7th
Eighth	8th
Ninth	9th
Tenth	10th
Eleventh	11th
Twelfth	12th
Thirteenth	13th
Fourteenth	14th
Fifteenth	15th
Sixteenth	16th
Seventeenth	17th
Eighteenth	18th
Nineteenth	19th
Twentieth	20th
Twenty-first	21st
Twenty-second	22d or 22nd
Twenty-third	23d or 23rd
Twenty-fourth	24th
Twenty-fifth	25th
Twenty-sixth	26th
Twenty-seventh	27th
Twenty-eighth	28th
Twenty-ninth	29th
Thirtieth	30th
Thirty-first	31st
Thirty-second	32d or 32nd
Fortieth	40th
Forty-first	41st
Forty-second	42d or 42nd
Fiftieth	50th
Sixtieth	60th
Seventieth	70th
Eightieth	80th
Ninetieth	90th
Hundredth or one hundredth	100th
Hundred and first or one hundred and first	101st
Hundred and second	102d or 102nd
Two hundredth	200th
Three hundredth	300th
Four hundredth	400th
Five hundredth	500th
Six hundredth	600th
Seven hundredth	700th

Name	Symbol
Eight hundredth	800th
Nine hundredth	900th
Thousandth or one thousandth	1000th
Two thousandth	2000th
Ten thousandth	10,000th
Hundred thousandth or one hundred thousandth	100,000th
Millionth or one millionth	1,000,000th

Denominations above one million

Name	Value in powers of ten	Number of zeros
American system		
Billion	10^9	9
Trillion	10^{12}	12
Quadrillion	10^{15}	15
Quintillion	10^{18}	18
Sextillion	10^{21}	21
Septillion	10^{24}	24
Octillion	10^{27}	27
Nonillion	10^{30}	30
Decillion	10^{33}	33
Undecillion	10^{36}	36
Duodecillion	10^{39}	39
Tredecillion	10^{42}	42
Quattuordecillion	10^{45}	45
Quindecillion	10^{48}	48
Sexdecillion	10^{51}	51
Septendecillion	10^{54}	54
Octodecillion	10^{57}	57
Novemdecillion	10^{60}	60
Vigintillion	10^{63}	63
Centillion	10^{303}	303
British system		
Milliard	10^9	9
Billion	10^{12}	12
Trillion	10^{18}	18
Quadrillion	10^{24}	24
Quintillion	10^{30}	30
Sextillion	10^{36}	36
Septillion	10^{42}	42
Octillion	10^{48}	48
Nonillion	10^{54}	54
Decillion	10^{60}	60
Undecillion	10^{66}	66
Duodecillion	10^{72}	72
Tredecillion	10^{78}	78
Quattuordecillion	10^{84}	84
Quindecillion	10^{90}	90
Sexdecillion	10^{96}	96
Septendecillion	10^{102}	102
Octodecillion	10^{108}	108
Novemdecillion	10^{114}	114
Vigintillion	10^{120}	120
Centillion	10^{600}	600

Four-place logarithms

N	0	1	2	3	4	5	6	7	8	9	Proportional Parts 1 2 3 4 5 6 7 8 9
10	0000	0043	0086	0128	0170	0212	0253	0294	0334	0374	*4 8 12 17 21 25 29 33 37
11	0414	0453	0492	0531	0569	0607	0645	0682	0719	0755	4 8 11 15 19 23 26 30 34
12	0792	0828	0864	0899	0934	0969	1004	1038	1072	1106	3 7 10 14 17 21 24 28 31
13	1139	1173	1206	1239	1271	1303	1335	1367	1399	1430	3 6 10 13 16 19 23 26 29
14	1461	1492	1523	1553	1584	1614	1644	1673	1703	1732	3 6 9 12 15 18 21 24 27
15	1761	1790	1818	1847	1875	1903	1931	1959	1987	2014	*3 6 8 11 14 17 20 22 25
16	2041	2068	2095	2122	2148	2175	2201	2227	2253	2279	3 5 8 11 13 16 18 21 24
17	2304	2330	2355	2380	2405	2430	2455	2480	2504	2529	2 5 7 10 12 15 17 20 22
18	2553	2577	2601	2625	2648	2672	2695	2718	2742	2765	2 5 7 9 12 14 16 19 21
19	2788	2810	2833	2856	2878	2900	2923	2945	2967	2989	2 4 7 9 11 13 16 18 20
20	3010	3032	3054	3075	3096	3118	3139	3160	3181	3201	2 4 6 8 11 13 15 17 19
21	3222	3243	3263	3284	3304	3324	3345	3365	3385	3404	2 4 6 8 10 12 14 16 18
22	3424	3444	3464	3483	3502	3522	3541	3560	3579	3598	2 4 6 8 10 12 14 15 17
23	3617	3636	3655	3674	3692	3711	3729	3747	3766	3784	2 4 6 7 9 11 13 15 17
24	3802	3820	3838	3856	3874	3892	3909	3927	3945	3962	2 4 5 7 9 11 12 14 16
25	3979	3997	4014	4031	4048	4065	4082	4099	4116	4133	2 3 5 7 9 10 12 14 15
26	4150	4166	4183	4200	4216	4232	4249	4265	4281	4298	2 3 5 7 8 10 11 13 15
27	4314	4330	4346	4362	4378	4393	4409	4425	4440	4456	2 3 5 6 8 9 11 13 14
28	4472	4487	4502	4518	4533	4548	4564	4579	4594	4609	2 3 5 6 8 9 11 12 14
29	4624	4639	4654	4669	4683	4698	4713	4728	4742	4757	1 3 4 6 7 9 10 12 13
30	4771	4786	4800	4814	4829	4843	4857	4871	4886	4900	1 3 4 6 7 9 10 11 13
31	4914	4928	4942	4955	4969	4983	4997	5011	5024	5038	1 3 4 6 7 8 10 11 12
32	5051	5065	5079	5092	5105	5119	5132	5145	5159	5172	1 3 4 5 7 8 9 11 12
33	5185	5198	5211	5224	5237	5250	5263	5276	5289	5302	1 3 4 5 6 8 9 10 12
34	5315	5328	5340	5353	5366	5378	5391	5403	5416	5428	1 3 4 5 6 8 9 10 11
35	5441	5453	5465	5478	5490	5502	5514	5527	5539	5551	1 2 4 5 6 7 9 10 11
36	5563	5575	5587	5599	5611	5623	5635	5647	5658	5670	1 2 4 5 6 7 8 10 11
37	5682	5694	5705	5717	5729	5740	5752	5763	5775	5786	1 2 3 5 6 7 8 9 10
38	5798	5809	5821	5832	5843	5855	5866	5877	5888	5899	1 2 3 5 6 7 8 9 10
39	5911	5922	5933	5944	5955	5966	5977	5988	5999	6010	1 2 3 4 5 7 8 9 10
40	6021	6031	6042	6053	6064	6075	6085	6096	6107	6117	1 2 3 4 5 6 8 9 10
41	6128	6138	6149	6160	6170	6180	6191	6201	6212	6222	1 2 3 4 5 6 7 8 9
42	6232	6243	6253	6263	6274	6284	6294	6304	6314	6325	1 2 3 4 5 6 7 8 9
43	6335	6345	6355	6365	6375	6385	6395	6405	6415	6425	1 2 3 4 5 6 7 8 9
44	6435	6444	6454	6464	6474	6484	6493	6503	6513	6522	1 2 3 4 5 6 7 8 9
45	6532	6542	6551	6561	6571	6580	6590	6599	6609	6618	1 2 3 4 5 6 7 8 9
46	6628	6637	6646	6656	6665	6675	6684	6693	6702	6712	1 2 3 4 5 6 7 7 8
47	6721	6730	6739	6749	6758	6767	6776	6785	6794	6803	1 2 3 4 5 5 6 7 8
48	6812	6821	6830	6839	6848	6857	6866	6875	6884	6893	1 2 3 4 4 5 6 7 8
49	6902	6911	6920	6928	6937	6946	6955	6964	6972	6981	1 2 3 4 4 5 6 7 8
50	6990	6998	7007	7016	7024	7033	7042	7050	7059	7067	1 2 3 3 4 5 6 7 8
51	7076	7084	7093	7101	7110	7118	7126	7135	7143	7152	1 2 3 3 4 5 6 7 8
52	7160	7168	7177	7185	7193	7202	7210	7218	7226	7235	1 2 2 3 4 5 6 7 7
53	7243	7251	7259	7267	7275	7284	7292	7300	7308	7316	1 2 2 3 4 5 6 6 7
54	7324	7332	7340	7348	7356	7364	7372	7380	7388	7396	1 2 2 3 4 5 6 6 7
N	0	1	2	3	4	5	6	7	8	9	1 2 3 4 5 6 7 8 9

*Interpolation in this section of the table is inaccurate. From Handbook of chemistry and physics, ed. 46, Weast, R. C., editor, 1965. Used by permission of CRC Press, Inc.

Continued.

N	0	1	2	3	4	5	6	7	8	9	Proportional Parts 1	2	3	4	5	6	7	8	9
55	7404	7412	7419	7427	7435	7443	7451	7459	7466	7474	1	2	2	3	4	5	5	6	7
56	7482	7490	7497	7505	7513	7520	7528	7536	7543	7551	1	2	2	3	4	5	5	6	7
57	7559	7566	7574	7582	7589	7597	7604	7612	7619	7627	1	2	2	3	4	5	5	6	7
58	7634	7642	7649	7657	7664	7672	7679	7686	7694	7701	1	1	2	3	4	4	5	6	7
59	7709	7716	7723	7731	7738	7745	7752	7760	7767	7774	1	1	2	3	4	4	5	6	7
60	7782	7789	7796	7803	7810	7818	7825	7832	7839	7846	1	1	2	3	4	4	5	6	6
61	7853	7860	7868	7875	7882	7889	7896	7903	7910	7917	1	1	2	3	4	4	5	6	6
62	7924	7931	7938	7945	7952	7959	7966	7973	7980	7987	1	1	2	3	3	4	5	6	6
63	7993	8000	8007	8014	8021	8028	8035	8041	8048	8055	1	1	2	3	3	4	5	5	6
64	8062	8069	8075	8082	8089	8096	8102	8109	8116	8122	1	1	2	3	3	4	5	5	6
65	8129	8136	8142	8149	8156	8162	8169	8176	8182	8189	1	1	2	3	3	4	5	5	6
66	8195	8202	8209	8215	8222	8228	8235	8241	8248	8254	1	1	2	3	3	4	5	5	6
67	8261	8267	8274	8280	8287	8293	8299	8306	8312	8319	1	1	2	3	3	4	5	5	6
68	8325	8331	8338	8344	8351	8357	8363	8370	8376	8382	1	1	2	3	3	4	4	5	6
69	8388	8395	8401	8407	8414	8420	8426	8432	8439	8445	1	1	2	2	3	4	4	5	6
70	8451	8457	8463	8470	8476	8482	8488	8494	8500	8506	1	1	2	2	3	4	4	5	6
71	8513	8519	8525	8531	8537	8543	8549	8555	8561	8567	1	1	2	2	3	4	4	5	5
72	8573	8579	8585	8591	8597	8603	8609	8615	8621	8627	1	1	2	2	3	4	4	5	5
73	8633	8639	8645	8651	8657	8663	8669	8675	8681	8686	1	1	2	2	3	4	4	5	5
74	8692	8698	8704	8710	8716	8722	8727	8733	8739	8745	1	1	2	2	3	4	4	5	5
75	8751	8756	8762	8768	8774	8779	8785	8791	8797	8802	1	1	2	2	3	3	4	5	5
76	8808	8814	8820	8825	8831	8837	8842	8848	8854	8859	1	1	2	2	3	3	4	5	5
77	8865	8871	8876	8882	8887	8893	8899	8904	8910	8915	1	1	2	2	3	3	4	4	5
78	8921	8927	8932	8938	8943	8949	8954	8960	8965	8971	1	1	2	2	3	3	4	4	5
79	8976	8982	8987	8993	8998	9004	9009	9015	9020	9025	1	1	2	2	3	3	4	4	5
80	9031	9036	9042	9047	9053	9058	9063	9069	9074	9079	1	1	2	2	3	3	4	4	5
81	9085	9090	9096	9101	9106	9112	9117	9122	9128	9133	1	1	2	2	3	3	4	4	5
82	9138	9143	9149	9154	9159	9165	9170	9175	9180	9186	1	1	2	2	3	3	4	4	5
83	9191	9196	9201	9206	9212	9217	9222	9227	9232	9238	1	1	2	2	3	3	4	4	5
84	9243	9248	9253	9258	9263	9269	9274	9279	9284	9289	1	1	2	2	3	3	4	4	5
85	9294	9299	9304	9309	9315	9320	9325	9330	9335	9340	1	1	2	2	3	3	4	4	5
86	9345	9350	9355	9360	9365	9370	9375	9380	9385	9390	1	1	2	2	3	3	4	4	5
87	9395	9400	9405	9410	9415	9420	9425	9430	9435	9440	0	1	1	2	2	3	3	4	4
88	9445	9450	9455	9460	9465	9469	9474	9479	9484	9489	0	1	1	2	2	3	3	4	4
89	9494	9499	9504	9509	9513	9518	9523	9528	9533	9538	0	1	1	2	2	3	3	4	4
90	9542	9547	9552	9557	9562	9566	9571	9576	9581	9586	0	1	1	2	2	3	3	4	4
91	9590	9595	9600	9605	9609	9614	9619	9624	9628	9633	0	1	1	2	2	3	3	4	4
92	9638	9643	9647	9652	9657	9661	9666	9671	9675	9680	0	1	1	2	2	3	3	4	4
93	9685	9689	9694	9699	9703	9708	9713	9717	9722	9727	0	1	1	2	2	3	3	4	4
94	9731	9736	9741	9745	9750	9754	9759	9763	9768	9773	0	1	1	2	2	3	3	4	4
95	9777	9782	9786	9791	9795	9800	9805	9809	9814	9818	0	1	1	2	2	3	3	4	4
96	9823	9827	9832	9836	9841	9845	9850	9854	9859	9863	0	1	1	2	2	3	3	4	4
97	9868	9872	9877	9881	9886	9890	9894	9899	9903	9908	0	1	1	2	2	3	3	4	4
98	9912	9917	9921	9926	9930	9934	9939	9943	9948	9952	0	1	1	2	2	3	3	4	4
99	9956	9961	9965	9969	9974	9978	9983	9987	9991	9996	0	1	1	2	2	3	3	3	4
N	0	1	2	3	4	5	6	7	8	9	1	2	3	4	5	6	7	8	9

Antilogarithms

	0	1	2	3	4	5	6	7	8	9	Proportional Parts								
											1	2	3	4	5	6	7	8	9
.00	1000	1002	1005	1007	1009	1012	1014	1016	1019	1021	0	0	1	1	1	1	2	2	2
.01	1023	1026	1028	1030	1033	1035	1038	1040	1042	1045	0	0	1	1	1	1	2	2	2
.02	1047	1050	1052	1054	1057	1059	1062	1064	1067	1069	0	0	1	1	1	1	2	2	2
.03	1072	1074	1076	1079	1081	1084	1086	1089	1091	1094	0	0	1	1	1	1	2	2	2
.04	1096	1099	1102	1104	1107	1109	1112	1114	1117	1119	0	1	1	1	1	2	2	2	2
.05	1122	1125	1127	1130	1132	1135	1138	1140	1143	1146	0	1	1	1	1	2	2	2	2
.06	1148	1151	1153	1156	1159	1161	1164	1167	1169	1172	0	1	1	1	1	2	2	2	2
.07	1175	1178	1180	1183	1186	1189	1191	1194	1197	1199	0	1	1	1	1	2	2	2	2
.08	1202	1205	1208	1211	1213	1216	1219	1222	1225	1227	0	1	1	1	1	2	2	2	3
.09	1230	1233	1236	1239	1242	1245	1247	1250	1253	1256	0	1	1	1	1	2	2	2	3
.10	1259	1262	1265	1268	1271	1274	1276	1279	1282	1285	0	1	1	1	1	2	2	2	3
.11	1288	1291	1294	1297	1300	1303	1306	1309	1312	1315	0	1	1	1	2	2	2	3	3
.12	1318	1321	1324	1327	1330	1334	1337	1340	1343	1346	0	1	1	1	2	2	2	3	3
.13	1349	1352	1355	1358	1361	1365	1368	1371	1374	1377	0	1	1	1	2	2	2	3	3
.14	1380	1384	1387	1390	1393	1396	1400	1403	1406	1409	0	1	1	1	2	2	2	3	3
.15	1413	1416	1419	1422	1426	1429	1432	1435	1439	1442	0	1	1	1	2	2	2	3	3
.16	1445	1449	1452	1455	1459	1462	1466	1469	1472	1476	0	1	1	1	2	2	2	3	3
.17	1479	1483	1486	1489	1493	1496	1500	1503	1507	1510	0	1	1	1	2	2	2	3	3
.18	1514	1517	1521	1524	1528	1531	1535	1538	1542	1545	0	1	1	1	2	2	2	3	3
.19	1549	1552	1556	1560	1563	1567	1570	1574	1578	1581	0	1	1	1	2	2	3	3	3
.20	1585	1589	1592	1596	1600	1603	1607	1611	1614	1618	0	1	1	1	2	2	3	3	3
.21	1622	1626	1629	1633	1637	1641	1644	1648	1652	1656	0	1	1	2	2	2	3	3	3
.22	1660	1663	1667	1671	1675	1679	1683	1687	1690	1694	0	1	1	2	2	2	3	3	3
.23	1698	1702	1706	1710	1714	1718	1722	1726	1730	1734	0	1	1	2	2	2	3	3	4
.24	1738	1742	1746	1750	1754	1758	1762	1766	1770	1774	0	1	1	2	2	2	3	3	4
.25	1778	1782	1786	1791	1795	1799	1803	1807	1811	1816	0	1	1	2	2	2	3	3	4
.26	1820	1824	1828	1832	1837	1841	1845	1849	1854	1858	0	1	1	2	2	3	3	3	4
.27	1862	1866	1871	1875	1879	1884	1888	1892	1897	1901	0	1	1	2	2	3	3	3	4
.28	1905	1910	1914	1919	1923	1928	1932	1936	1941	1945	0	1	1	2	2	3	3	4	4
.29	1950	1954	1959	1963	1968	1972	1977	1982	1986	1991	0	1	1	2	2	3	3	4	4
.30	1995	2000	2004	2009	2014	2018	2023	2028	2032	2037	0	1	1	2	2	3	3	4	4
.31	2042	2046	2051	2056	2061	2065	2070	2075	2080	2084	0	1	1	2	2	3	3	4	4
.32	2089	2094	2099	2104	2109	2113	2118	2123	2128	2133	0	1	1	2	2	3	3	4	4
.33	2138	2143	2148	2153	2158	2163	2168	2173	2178	2183	0	1	1	2	2	3	3	4	4
.34	2188	2193	2198	2203	2208	2213	2218	2223	2228	2234	1	1	2	2	3	3	4	4	5
.35	2239	2244	2249	2254	2259	2265	2270	2275	2280	2286	1	1	2	2	3	3	4	4	5
.36	2291	2296	2301	2307	2312	2317	2323	2328	2333	2339	1	1	2	2	3	3	4	4	5
.37	2344	2350	2355	2360	2366	2371	2377	2382	2388	2393	1	1	2	2	3	3	4	4	5
.38	2399	2404	2410	2415	2421	2427	2432	2438	2443	2449	1	1	2	2	3	3	4	5	5
.39	2455	2460	2466	2472	2477	2483	2489	2495	2500	2506	1	1	2	2	3	3	4	5	5
.40	2512	2518	2523	2529	2535	2541	2547	2553	2559	2564	1	1	2	2	3	4	4	5	5
.41	2570	2576	2582	2588	2594	2600	2606	2612	2618	2624	1	1	2	2	3	4	4	5	5
.42	2630	2636	2642	2649	2655	2661	2667	2673	2679	2685	1	1	2	2	3	4	4	5	6
.43	2692	2698	2704	2710	2716	2723	2729	2735	2742	2748	1	1	2	3	3	4	4	5	6
.44	2754	2761	2767	2773	2780	2786	2793	2799	2805	2812	1	1	2	3	3	4	4	5	6
.45	2818	2825	2831	2838	2844	2851	2858	2864	2871	2877	1	1	2	3	3	4	5	5	6
.46	2884	2891	2897	2904	2911	2917	2924	2931	2938	2944	1	1	2	3	3	4	5	5	6
.47	2951	2958	2965	2972	2979	2985	2992	2999	3006	3013	1	1	2	3	3	4	5	5	6
.48	3020	3027	3034	3041	3048	3055	3062	3069	3076	3083	1	1	2	3	4	4	5	6	6
.49	3090	3097	3105	3112	3119	3126	3133	3141	3148	3155	1	1	2	3	4	4	5	6	6
	0	1	2	3	4	5	6	7	8	9	1	2	3	4	5	6	7	8	9

From Handbook of chemistry and physics, ed. 46, Weast, R. C., editor, 1965. Used by permission of CRC Press, Inc. *Continued.*

	0	1	2	3	4	5	6	7	8	9	Proportional Parts 1	2	3	4	5	6	7	8	9
.50	3162	3170	3177	3184	3192	3199	3206	3214	3221	3228	1	1	2	3	4	4	5	6	7
.51	3236	3243	3251	3258	3266	3273	3281	3289	3296	3304	1	2	2	3	4	5	5	6	7
.52	3311	3319	3327	3334	3342	3350	3357	3365	3373	3381	1	2	2	3	4	5	5	6	7
.53	3388	3396	3404	3412	3420	3428	3436	3443	3451	3459	1	2	2	3	4	5	6	6	7
.54	3467	3475	3483	3491	3499	3508	3516	3524	3532	3540	1	2	2	3	4	5	6	6	7
.55	3548	3556	3565	3573	3581	3589	3597	3606	3614	3622	1	2	2	3	4	5	6	7	7
.56	3631	3639	3648	3656	3664	3673	3681	3690	3698	3707	1	2	3	3	4	5	6	7	8
.57	3715	3724	3733	3741	3750	3758	3767	3776	3784	3793	1	2	3	3	4	5	6	7	8
.58	3802	3811	3819	3828	3837	3846	3855	3864	3873	3882	1	2	3	4	4	5	6	7	8
.59	3890	3899	3908	3917	3926	3936	3945	3954	3963	3972	1	2	3	4	5	5	6	7	8
.60	3981	3990	3999	4009	4018	4027	4036	4046	4055	4064	1	2	3	4	5	6	6	7	8
.61	4074	4083	4093	4102	4111	4121	4130	4140	4150	4159	1	2	3	4	5	6	7	8	9
.62	4169	4178	4188	4198	4207	4217	4227	4236	4246	4256	1	2	3	4	5	6	7	8	9
.63	4266	4276	4285	4295	4305	4315	4325	4335	4345	4355	1	2	3	4	5	6	7	8	9
.64	4365	4375	4385	4395	4406	4416	4426	4436	4446	4457	1	2	3	4	5	6	7	8	9
.65	4467	4477	4487	4498	4508	4519	4529	4539	4550	4560	1	2	3	4	5	6	7	8	9
.66	4571	4581	4592	4603	4613	4624	4634	4645	4656	4667	1	2	3	4	5	6	7	9	10
.67	4677	4688	4699	4710	4721	4732	4742	4753	4764	4775	1	2	3	4	5	7	8	9	10
.68	4786	4797	4808	4819	4831	4842	4853	4864	4875	4887	1	2	3	4	6	7	8	9	10
.69	4898	4909	4920	4932	4943	4955	4966	4977	4989	5000	1	2	3	5	6	7	8	9	10
.70	5012	5023	5035	5047	5058	5070	5082	5093	5105	5117	1	2	4	5	6	7	8	9	11
.71	5129	5140	5152	5164	5176	5188	5200	5212	5224	5236	1	2	4	5	6	7	8	10	11
.72	5248	5260	5272	5284	5297	5309	5321	5333	5346	5358	1	2	4	5	6	7	9	10	11
.73	5370	5383	5395	5408	5420	5433	5445	5458	5470	5483	1	3	4	5	6	8	9	10	11
.74	5495	5508	5521	5534	5546	5559	5572	5585	5598	5610	1	3	4	5	6	8	9	10	12
.75	5623	5636	5649	5662	5675	5689	5702	5715	5728	5741	1	3	4	5	7	8	9	10	12
.76	5754	5768	5781	5794	5808	5821	5834	5848	5861	5875	1	3	4	5	7	8	9	11	12
.77	5888	5902	5916	5929	5943	5957	5970	5984	5998	6012	1	3	4	5	7	8	10	11	12
.78	6026	6039	6053	6067	6081	6095	6109	6124	6138	6152	1	3	4	6	7	8	10	11	13
.79	6166	6180	6194	6209	6223	6237	6252	6266	6281	6295	1	3	4	6	7	9	10	11	13
.80	6310	6324	6339	6353	6368	6383	6397	6412	6427	6442	1	3	4	6	7	9	10	12	13
.81	6457	6471	6486	6501	6516	6531	6546	6561	6577	6592	2	3	5	6	8	9	11	12	14
.82	6607	6622	6637	6653	6668	6683	6699	6714	6730	6745	2	3	5	6	8	9	11	12	14
.83	6761	6776	6792	6808	6823	6839	6855	6871	6887	6902	2	3	5	6	8	9	11	13	14
.84	6918	6934	6950	6966	6982	6998	7015	7031	7047	7063	2	3	5	6	8	10	11	13	15
.85	7079	7096	7112	7129	7145	7161	7178	7194	7211	7228	2	3	5	7	8	10	12	13	15
.86	7244	7261	7278	7295	7311	7328	7345	7362	7379	7396	2	3	5	7	8	10	12	13	15
.87	7413	7430	7447	7464	7482	7499	7516	7534	7551	7568	2	3	5	7	9	10	12	14	16
.88	7586	7603	7621	7638	7656	7674	7691	7709	7727	7745	2	4	5	7	9	11	12	14	16
.89	7762	7780	7798	7816	7834	7852	7870	7889	7907	7925	2	4	5	7	9	11	13	14	16
.90	7943	7962	7980	7998	8017	8035	8054	8072	8091	8110	2	4	6	7	9	11	13	15	17
.91	8128	8147	8166	8185	8204	8222	8241	8260	8279	8299	2	4	6	8	9	11	13	15	17
.92	8318	8337	8356	8375	8395	8414	8433	8453	8472	8492	2	4	6	8	10	12	14	15	17
.93	8511	8531	8551	8570	8590	8610	8630	8650	8670	8690	2	4	6	8	10	12	14	16	18
.94	8710	8730	8750	8770	8790	8810	8831	8851	8872	8892	2	4	6	8	10	12	14	16	18
.95	8913	8933	8954	8974	8995	9016	9036	9057	9078	9099	2	4	6	8	10	12	15	17	19
.96	9120	9141	9162	9183	9204	9226	9247	9268	9290	9311	2	4	6	8	11	13	15	17	19
.97	9333	9354	9376	9397	9419	9441	9462	9484	9506	9528	2	4	7	9	11	13	15	17	20
.98	9550	9572	9594	9616	9638	9661	9683	9705	9727	9750	2	4	7	9	11	13	16	18	20
.99	9772	9795	9817	9840	9863	9886	9908	9931	9954	9977	2	5	7	9	11	14	16	18	20
	0	1	2	3	4	5	6	7	8	9	1	2	3	4	5	6	7	8	9

Square root chart for calculating standard deviation $SD = \sqrt{\dfrac{\sum(X-\bar{X})^2}{n-1}}$

The columns designated with the square root sign $\sqrt{}$ are the numbers for which the square root is to be determined. The column to the right contains the number that is the square root value (or SD). For example, the square root of 1.2 is 1.09 (1.09 $\times$ 1.09 = 1.2). The square root of 5 is 2.24 the square root of 10.8 is 3.29. To determine square roots of numbers from 0.01 to 0.099 and from 0.10 to 0.99.

1. Move decimal point two places to right (0.02 becomes 2.0).
2. Move decimal point of numbers next to the square root column one place to left (1.41 becomes 0.141).

EXAMPLE: What is the square root of 0.02?

1. Move decimal two places to right = 2.0.
2. Opposite 2.0 find the square root number 1.41.
3. Move decimal point one place to left (1.41 becomes 0.141).
4. Square root of 0.02 ($\sqrt{0.02}$) is 0.141.

EXAMPLE: What is the square root of 0.96?

1. Move decimal point two places to right (0.96 becomes 96).
2. Opposite 96 to 9.80.
3. Move decimal point one place to left (9.80 becomes 0.98).
4. Square root of 0.96 ($\sqrt{0.96}$) is 0.98.

EXAMPLE: Using the above system for calculating standard deviation as applied to 10 calcium determinations on the same sample.

Number of tests	Values A (X)	Difference from mean B ($\bar{X}$-X)	Difference from mean squared C ($\bar{X}$-X)^2
1	9.8	(10 − 9.8) = 0.2	(0.2 × 0.2) = 0.04
2	10.2	0.2	0.04
3	9.9	0.1	0.01
4	10.1	0.1	0.01
5	9.7	0.3	0.09
6	10.3	0.3	0.09
7	10.0	0.0	0.00
8	10.0	0.0	0.00
9	9.9	0.1	0.01
10	10.1	0.1	0.01
	100.0		0.30

Average (mean) = $\dfrac{100.0}{10}$ = 10

$\dfrac{0.30}{(10 - 1) \text{ or } 9}$ $\dfrac{\text{Sum of differences squared (column } C)}{\text{Number of tests less 1}}$ = 0.033

To calculate square root of 0.033

1. Move decimal point two places to right (0.033 becomes 3.3).
2. From square root chart, next to 3.3 find number that is square root (take average between 3.2 and 3.4 = 1.815).
3. Square root of 3.3 is 1.815.
4. Move decimal point one place to left (1.815 becomes 0.1815 or 0.18).
5. Therefore, square root of 0.033 is 0.18.
6. 1 SD = ±0.18   2 SD = ±0.36   3 SD = ±0.54

Square roots of numbers from 1 to 100 in steps of 0.2

	SD		SD		SD		SD		SD
$\sqrt{1.0}$	1.00	$\sqrt{11}$	3.32	$\sqrt{21}$	4.58	$\sqrt{31}$	5.57	$\sqrt{41}$	6.40
1.2	1.09	11.2	3.35	21.2	4.60	31.2	5.59	41.2	6.42
1.4	1.18	11.4	3.38	21.4	4.63	31.4	5.60	41.4	6.43
1.6	1.26	11.6	3.41	21.6	4.65	31.6	5.62	41.6	6.45
1.8	1.34	11.8	3.44	21.8	4.67	31.8	5.64	41.8	6.47
2.0	1.41	12	3.46	22	4.69	32	5.66	42	6.48
2.2	1.48	12.2	3.49	22.2	4.71	32.2	5.67	42.2	6.50
2.4	1.55	12.4	3.52	22.4	4.73	32.4	5.69	42.4	6.51
2.6	1.61	12.6	3.55	22.6	4.75	32.6	5.71	42.6	6.53
2.8	1.67	12.8	3.58	22.8	4.77	32.8	5.73	42.8	6.54
3.0	1.73	13	3.61	23	4.80	33	5.74	43	6.56
3.2	1.79	13.2	3.63	23.2	4.82	33.2	5.76	43.2	6.57
3.4	1.84	13.4	3.66	23.4	4.84	33.4	5.78	43.4	6.59
3.6	1.90	13.6	3.69	23.6	4.86	33.6	5.80	43.6	6.60
3.8	1.95	13.8	3.71	23.8	4.88	33.8	5.81	43.8	6.62
4.0	2.0	14	3.74	24	4.90	34	5.83	44	6.63
4.2	2.05	14.2	3.77	24.2	4.92	34.2	5.85	44.2	6.65
4.4	2.10	14.4	3.79	24.4	4.94	34.4	5.87	44.4	6.66
4.6	2.14	14.6	3.82	24.6	4.96	34.6	5.88	44.6	6.68
4.8	2.19	14.8	3.85	24.8	4.98	34.8	5.90	44.8	6.69
5.0	2.24	15	3.87	25	5.00	35	5.92	45	6.71
5.2	2.28	15.2	3.90	25.2	5.02	35.2	5.93	45.2	6.72
5.4	2.32	15.4	3.92	25.4	5.04	35.4	5.95	45.4	6.74
5.6	2.37	15.6	3.95	25.6	5.06	35.6	5.97	45.6	6.75
5.8	2.41	15.8	3.97	25.8	5.08	35.8	5.98	45.8	6.77
6.0	2.45	16	4.00	26	5.10	36	6.00	46	6.78
6.2	2.49	16.2	4.02	26.2	5.12	36.2	6.02	46.2	6.80
6.4	2.53	16.4	4.05	26.4	5.14	36.4	6.03	46.4	6.81
6.6	2.57	16.6	4.07	26.6	5.16	36.6	6.05	46.6	6.83
6.8	2.61	16.8	4.10	26.8	5.18	36.8	6.07	46.8	6.84
7.0	2.65	17	4.12	27	5.20	37	6.08	47	6.86
7.2	2.68	17.2	4.15	27.2	5.22	37.2	6.10	47.2	6.87
7.4	2.72	17.4	4.17	27.4	5.23	37.4	6.12	47.4	6.88
7.6	2.76	17.6	4.20	27.6	5.25	37.6	6.13	47.6	6.90
7.8	2.79	17.8	4.22	27.8	5.27	37.8	6.15	47.8	6.91
8.0	2.83	18	4.24	28	5.29	38	6.16	48	6.93
8.2	2.86	18.2	4.27	28.2	5.31	38.2	6.18	48.2	6.94
8.4	2.90	18.4	4.29	28.4	5.33	38.4	6.20	48.4	6.96
8.6	2.93	18.6	4.31	28.6	5.35	38.6	6.21	48.6	6.97
8.8	2.97	18.8	4.34	28.8	5.37	38.8	6.23	48.8	6.99
9.0	3.0	19	4.36	29	5.39	39	6.24	49	7.00
9.2	3.03	19.2	4.38	29.2	5.50	39.2	6.26	49.2	7.01
9.4	3.07	19.4	4.40	29.4	5.42	39.4	6.28	49.4	7.03
9.6	3.10	19.6	4.43	29.6	5.44	39.6	6.29	49.6	7.04
9.8	3.13	19.8	4.45	29.8	5.46	39.8	6.31	49.8	7.06
10	3.16	20	4.47	30	5.48	40	6.32	50	7.07
10.2	3.19	20.2	4.49	30.2	5.50	40.2	6.34	50.2	7.09
10.4	3.22	20.4	4.52	30.4	5.51	40.4	6.36	50.4	7.10
10.6	3.26	20.6	4.54	30.6	5.53	40.6	6.37	50.6	7.11
10.8	3.29	20.8	4.56	30.8	5.55	40.8	6.39	50.8	7.13

Used with permission of DADE Div AHSC Miami, Fla.

	SD		SD		SD		SD		SD
$\sqrt{51}$	7.14	$\sqrt{61}$	7.81	$\sqrt{71}$	8.43	$\sqrt{81}$	9.00	$\sqrt{91}$	9.54
51.2	7.16	61.2	7.82	71.2	8.44	81.2	9.01	91.2	9.55
51.4	7.17	61.4	7.84	71.4	8.45	81.4	9.02	91.4	9.56
51.6	7.18	61.6	7.85	71.6	8.46	81.6	9.03	91.6	9.57
51.8	7.20	61.8	7.86	71.8	8.47	81.8	9.04	91.8	9.58
52	7.21	62	7.87	72	8.49	82	9.06	92	9.59
52.2	7.22	62.2	7.89	72.2	8.50	82.2	9.07	92.2	9.60
52.4	7.24	62.4	7.90	72.4	8.51	82.4	9.08	92.4	9.61
52.6	7.25	62.6	7.91	72.6	8.52	82.6	9.09	92.6	9.62
52.8	7.27	62.8	7.92	72.8	8.53	82.8	9.10	92.8	9.63
53	7.28	63	7.94	73	8.54	83	9.11	93	9.64
53.2	7.29	63.2	7.95	73.2	8.56	83.2	9.12	93.2	9.65
53.4	7.31	63.4	7.96	73.4	8.57	83.4	9.13	93.4	9.66
53.6	7.32	63.6	7.97	73.6	8.58	83.6	9.14	93.6	9.67
53.8	7.33	63.8	7.99	73.8	8.59	83.8	9.15	93.8	9.68
54	7.35	64	8.00	74	8.60	84	9.17	94	9.70
54.2	7.36	64.2	8.01	74.2	8.61	84.2	9.18	94.2	9.71
54.4	7.38	64.4	8.02	74.4	8.63	84.4	9.19	94.4	9.72
54.6	7.39	64.6	8.04	74.6	8.64	84.6	9.20	94.6	9.73
54.8	7.40	64.8	8.05	74.8	8.65	84.8	9.21	94.8	9.74
55	7.42	65	8.06	75	8.66	85	9.22	95	9.75
55.2	7.43	65.2	8.07	75.2	8.67	85.2	9.23	95.2	9.76
55.4	7.44	65.4	8.09	75.4	8.68	85.4	9.24	95.4	9.77
55.6	7.46	65.6	8.10	75.6	8.69	85.6	9.25	95.6	9.78
55.8	7.47	65.8	8.11	75.8	8.71	85.8	9.26	95.8	9.79
56	7.48	66	8.12	76	8.72	86	9.27	96	9.80
56.2	7.50	66.2	8.14	76.2	8.73	86.2	9.28	96.2	9.81
56.4	7.51	66.4	8.15	76.4	8.74	86.4	9.30	96.4	9.82
56.6	7.52	66.6	8.16	76.6	8.75	86.6	9.31	96.6	9.83
56.8	7.54	66.8	8.17	76.8	8.76	86.8	9.32	96.8	9.84
57	7.55	67	8.19	77	8.77	87	9.33	97	9.85
57.2	7.57	67.2	8.20	77.2	8.79	87.2	9.34	97.2	9.86
57.4	7.58	67.4	8.21	77.4	8.80	87.4	9.35	97.4	9.87
57.6	7.59	67.6	8.22	77.6	8.81	87.6	9.36	97.6	9.88
57.8	7.60	67.8	8.23	77.8	8.82	87.8	9.37	97.8	9.89
58	7.62	68	8.25	78	8.83	88	9.38	98	9.90
58.2	7.63	68.2	8.26	78.2	8.84	88.2	9.39	98.2	9.91
58.4	7.64	68.4	8.27	78.4	8.85	88.4	9.40	98.4	9.92
58.6	7.66	68.6	8.28	78.6	8.87	88.6	9.41	98.6	9.93
58.8	7.67	68.8	8.29	78.8	8.88	88.8	9.42	98.8	9.94
59	7.68	69	8.31	79	8.89	89	9.43	99	9.94
59.2	7.69	69.2	8.32	79.2	8.90	89.2	9.44	99.2	9.96
59.4	7.71	69.4	8.33	79.4	8.91	89.4	9.46	99.4	9.97
59.6	7.72	69.6	8.34	79.6	8.92	89.6	9.47	99.6	9.98
59.8	7.73	69.8	8.35	79.8	8.93	89.8	9.48	99.8	9.99
60	7.75	70	8.37	80	8.94	90	9.49		
60.2	7.76	70.2	8.38	80.2	8.96	90.2	9.50		
60.4	7.77	70.4	8.39	80.4	8.97	90.4	9.51		
60.6	7.78	70.6	8.40	80.6	8.98	90.6	9.52		
60.8	7.80	70.8	8.41	80.8	8.99	90.8	9.53		

Apothecary, avoirdupois, and troy systems of measure

The grain is the same in all three systems: 1 grain = 64.8 mg = 0.0648 gm.

1. Apothecaries' weight: A system of weights used in compounding prescriptions, based on the grain (64.8 mg) and the minim (0.061610 ml).

Dry	Liquid (U. S.)
Grain = 64.8 mg	Minim = 0.061610 ml
Scruple = 20 grains	Fluidram = 60 minims
Dram = 3 scruples	Fluidounce = 8 fluidrams
Ounce = 8 drams	Gill = 4 fluidounces
Pound = 12 ounces	Pint = 4 gills
	Quart = 2 pints
	Gallon = 4 quarts

2. Avoirdupois weight: The system of weight commonly used for ordinary commodities in English-speaking countries.

> Grain = 64.8 mg
> Dram = 27.344 grains
> Ounce = 16 drams
> Pound = 16 ounces

3. Troy weight: A system of weights used by jewelers for gold and precious stones.

> Grain = 64.8 mg
> Pennyweight = 24 grains
> Dram = 2.5 pennyweight = 60 grains
> Ounce = 20 pennyweight = 8 drams
> Pound = 12 ounces

Conversion factors for units of measure

To convert from unit	Abbreviation —symbol	To	Multiply by
Acres		Sq centimeters	40,468,564
		Sq feet	43,560
		Sq kilometers	0.0040468564
		Sq links (Gunter's)	1×10^5
		Sq meters	4046.8564
		Sq miles (statute)	0.0015625
		Sq rods	160
		Sq yards	4840
Ångström units	Å	Centimeters	1×10^{-8}
		Inches	3.9370079×10^{-9}
		Micrometers	0.0001
		Nanometers	0.1
Ares	a	Acres	0.024710538
		Sq dekameters	1
		Sq feet	1076.3910
		Sq feet (U. S. survey)	1076.3867
		Sq meters	100
		Sq miles	3.8610216×10^{-5}
Atmospheres	atm	Bars	1.01325
		cm Hg (0°C)	76
		cm H_2O (4°C)	1033.26
		Feet of H_2O (39.2°F)	33.8995
		Grams/sq centimeter	1033.23
		Inches of Hg (32°F)	29.9213
		Kilogram/sq centimeters	1.03323
		mm Hg (0°C)	760
		Pounds/sq inch	14.6960
		Torrs	760
Centigrams	cg	Grains	0.15432358
		Grams	0.01
Centiliters	cl	Cu centimeters	10
		Cu inches	0.6102545
		Liters	0.01
		Ounces (U. S., fluid)	0.3381497
Centimeters	cm	Ångström units	1×10^8
		Feet	0.032808399
		Inches	0.39370079
		Meters	0.01
		Microns	10,000
		Miles (naut., int.)	5.3995680×10^{-6}
		Miles (statute)	6.2137119×10^{-6}
		Millimeters	10
		Nanometers	1×10^7
		Rods	0.0019883878
		Yards	0.010936133

Modified from Weast, R. C., editor: Handbook of chemistry and physics, ed. 54, Cleveland, Ohio, 1973, CRC Press, Inc.

To convert from unit	Abbreviation —symbol	To	Multiply by
Cubic centimeters	cm³	Bushels (Brit.)	2.749617×10^{-5}
		Bushels (U. S.)	2.837759×10^{-5}
		Cu feet	3.5314667×10^{-5}
		Cu inches	0.061023744
		Cu meters	1×6^{-6}
		Cu yards	1.3079506×10^{-6}
		Drams (U. S., fluid)	0.27051218
		Gallons (Brit.)	0.0002199694
		Gallons (U. S., dry)	0.00022702075
		Gallons (U. S., liq.)	0.00026417205
		Gills (Brit.)	0.007039020
		Gills (U. S.)	0.0084535058
		Liters	0.001
		Ounces (Brit., fluid)	0.03519510
		Ounces (U. S., fluid)	0.033814023
		Pints (U. S., dry)	0.0018161660
		Pints (U. S., liq.)	0.0021133764
		Quarts (Brit.)	0.0008798775
		Quarts (U. S., dry)	0.00090808298
		Quarts (U. S., liq.)	0.0010566882
Cubic decimeters	dm³	Cu centimeters	1000
		Cu feet	0.035316667
		Cu inches	61.023744
		Cu meters	0.001
		Cu yards	0.0013079506
		Liters	1
Cubic dekameters	dkm³	Cu decimeters	1×10^{6}
		Cu feet	35,314.667
		Cu inches	6.1023744×10^{7}
		Cu meters	1000
		Liters	1,000,000
Cubic feet	ft³	Cu centimeters	28,316.847
		Cu meters	0.028316847
		Gallons (U. S., dry)	6.4285116
		Gallons (U. S., liq.)	7.4805195
		Liters	28.316847
		Ounces (Brit., fluid)	996.6143
		Ounces (U. S., fluid)	957.50649
		Pints (U. S., liq.)	59.844156
		Quarts (U. S., dry)	25.714047
		Quarts (U. S., liq.)	29.922078
Cubic inches	in³	Cu centimeters	16.387064
		Cu feet	0.00057870370
		Cu meters	1.6387064×10^{-5}
		Cu yards	2.1433470×10^{-5}
		Drams (U. S., fluid)	4.4329004
		Gallons (Brit.)	0.003604652
		Gallons (U. S., dry)	0.0037202035
		Gallons (U. S., liq.)	0.0043290043
		Liters	0.016387064
		Milliliters	16.387064

To convert from unit	Abbreviation —symbol	To	Multiply by
Cubic inches—cont'd		Ounces (Brit., fluid)	0.57674444
		Ounces (U. S., fluid)	0.55411255
		Pints (U. S., dry)	0.029761628
		Pints (U. S., liq.)	0.034632035
		Quarts (U. S., dry)	0.014880814
		Quarts (U. S., liq.)	0.017316017
Cubic meters	m^3	Cu centimeters	1×10^6
		Cu feet	35.314667
		Cu inches	61,023.74
		Cu yards	1.3079506
		Gallons (Brit.)	219.9694
		Gallons (U. S., liq.)	264.17205
		Liters	1000
		Pints (U. S., liq.)	2113.3764
		Quarts (U. S., liq.)	1056.6882
Cubic millimeters	mm^3	Cu centimeters	0.001
		Cu inches	6.1023744×10^{-5}
		Cu meters	1×10^{-9}
		Minims (Brit.)	0.01689365
		Minims (U. S.)	0.016230731
Decimeters	dm	Centimeters	10
		Feet	0.32808399
		Inches	3.9370079
		Meters	0.1
Dekaliters	dkl	Pecks (U. S.)	1.135136
		Pints (U. S., dry)	18.16217
Dekameters	dkm	Centimeters	1000
		Feet	32.808399
		Inches	393.70079
		Kilometers	0.01
		Meters	10
		Yards	10.93613
Drams (apoth. or troy)	dr ap ʒ	Drams (avdp.)	2.1942857
		Grains	60
		Grams	3887.9346
		Ounces (apoth. or troy)	0.125
		Ounces (avdp.)	0.13714286
		Scruples (apoth.)	3
Drams (avdp.)	dr avdp	Drams (apoth. or troy)	0.455729166
		Grains	27.34375
		Grams	1.7718452
		Ounces (apoth. or troy)	0.056966146
		Ounces (avdp.)	0.0625
		Pennyweights	1.1393229
		Pounds (apoth. or troy)	0.0047471788
		Pounds (avdp.)	0.00390625
		Scruples (apoth.)	1.3671875
Drams (U. S., fluid)	fl dr	Cu centimeters	3.6967162
		Cu inches	0.22558594

To convert from unit	Abbreviation —symbol	To	Multiply by
Drams (U. S., fluid)—cont'd		Gills (U. S.)	0.03125
		Milliliters	3.696588
		Minims (U. S.)	60
		Ounces (U. S., fluid)	0.125
		Pints (U. S., liq.)	0.0078125
Feet	ft	Centimeters	30.48
		Inches	12
		Meters	0.3048
		Microns	304,800
		Miles (naut., int.)	0.00016457883
		Miles (statute)	0.000189393
		Rods	0.060606
		Yards	0.333333
Firkins (Brit.)		Bushels (Brit.)	1.125
		Cu centimeters	40,914.79
		Cu feet	1.444892
		Firkins (U. S.)	1.200949
		Gallons (Brit.)	9
		Liters	40.91364
		Pints (Brit.)	72
Firkins (U. S.)		Barrels (U. S., dry)	0.29464286
		Barrels (U. S., liq.)	0.28571429
		Bushels (U. S.)	0.96678788
		Cu feet	1.203125
		Firkins (Brit.)	0.8326747
		Liters	34.06775
		Pints (U. S., liq.)	72
Gallons (Brit.)	gal	Barrels (Brit.)	0.027777
		Bushels (Brit.)	0.125
		Cu centimeters	4546.087
		Cu feet	0.1605436
		Cu inches	277.4193
		Firkins (Brit.)	0.111111
		Gallons (U. S., liq.)	1.200949
		Gills (Brit.)	32
		Liters	4.545960
		Minims (Brit.)	76,800
		Ounces (Brit., fluid)	160
		Ounces (U. S., fluid)	153.7215
		Pecks (Brit.)	0.5
		Pounds of H_2O (62°F)	10
Gallons (U. S., dry)		Barrels (U. S., dry)	0.038095592
		Barrels (U. S., liq.)	0.036941181
		Bushels (U. S.)	0.125
		Cu centimeters	4404.8828
		Cu feet	0.15555700
		Cu inches	268.8025
		Gallons (U. S., liq.)	1.16364719
		Liters	4.404760

To convert from units	Abbreviation —symbol	To	Multiply by
Gallons (U. S., liq.)	gal	Barrels (U. S., liq.)	0.031746032
		Bushels (U. S.)	0.10742088
		Cu centimeters	3785.4118
		Cu feet	0.13368055
		Cu inches	231
		Cu meters	0.0037854118
		Cu yards	0.0049511317
		Gallons (Brit.)	0.8326747
		Gallons (U. S., dry)	0.85936701
		Gallons (wine)	1
		Gills (U. S.)	32
		Liters	3.7854118
		Minims (U. S.)	61,440
		Ounces (U. S., fluid)	128
		Pints (U. S., liq.)	8
		Quarts (U. S., liq.)	4
Gills (Brit.)		Cu centimeters	142.0652
		Gallons (Brit.)	0.03125
		Gills (U. S.)	1.200949
		Liters	0.1420613
		Ounces (Brit., fluid)	5
		Ounces (U. S., fluid)	4.803764
		Pints (Brit.)	0.25
Gills (U. S.)		Cu centimeters	118.29412
		Cu inches	7.21875
		Drams (U. S., fluid)	32
		Gallons (U. S., liq.)	0.03125
		Gills (Brit.)	0.8326747
		Liters	0.1182908
		Minims (U. S.)	1920
		Ounces (U. S., fluid)	4
		Pints (U. S., liq.)	0.25
		Quarts (U. S., liq.)	0.125
Grains	gr	Carats (metric)	0.32399455
		Drams (apoth. or troy)	0.016666
		Drams (avdp.)	0.036571429
		Dynes	63.5460
		Grams	0.06479891
		Milligrams	64.79891
		Ounces (apoth. or troy)	0.0020833
		Ounces (avdp.)	0.002857143
		Pennyweights	0.041666
		Pounds (apoth. or troy)	0.000173611
		Pounds (avdp.)	0.00014285714
		Scruples (apoth.)	0.05
Grams	gm or g	Carats (metric)	5
		Decigrams	10
		Dekagrams	0.1
		Drams (apoth. or troy)	0.25720597
		Drams (avdp.)	0.56438339
		Grains	15.432358

To convert from unit	Abbreviation —symbol	To	Multiply by
Grams—cont'd		Kilograms	0.001
		Micrograms	1×10^6
		Myriagrams	0.0001
		Ounces (apoth. or troy)	0.32150737
		Ounces (avdp.)	0.35273962
		Pennyweights	0.64301493
		Poundals	0.0709316
		Pounds (apoth. or troy)	0.0026792289
		Pounds (avdp.)	0.0022046226
		Scruples (apoth.)	0.77161792
		Tons (metric)	1×10^{-6}
Hands		Centimeters	10.16
		Inches	4
Hectares	ha	Acres	2.4710538
		Ares	100
		Sq centimeters	1×10^8
		Sq feet	107,639.10
		Sq meters	10,000
		Sq miles	0.0038610216
		Sq rods	395.36861
Hectograms	hg	Grams	100
		Poundals	7.09316
		Pounds (apoth. or troy)	0.26792289
		Pounds (avdp.)	0.22046226
Hectoliters	hl	Bushels (Brit.)	2.749694
		Bushels (U. S.)	2.837839
		Cu centimeters	1.00028×10^5
		Cu feet	3.531566
		Gallons (U. S., liq.)	26.41794
		Liters	100
		Ounces (U. S., fluid)	3381.497
		Pecks (U. S.)	11.35136
Hectometers	hm	Centimeters	10,000
		Decimeters	1000
		Dekameters	10
		Feet	328.08399
		Meters	100
		Rods	19.883878
		Yards	109.3613
Inches	in	Ångström units	2.54×10^8
		Centimeters	2.54
		Cubits	0.055555
		Fathoms	0.013888
		Feet	0.083333
		Meters	0.0254
		Mils	1000
		Yards	0.027777
Inches of Hg (32°F)		Atmospheres	0.034211
		Bars	0.0338639
		Feet of air (1 atm, 60°F)	926.24

To convert from unit	Abbreviation —symbol	To	Multiply by
Inches of Hg (32°F)—cont'd		Feet of H_2O (39.2°F)	1.132957
		Grams/sq centimeter	34.5316
		Kilograms/sq meter	345.316
		Millimeters of Hg (60°C)	25.4
		Ounces/sq inch	7.85847
		Pounds/sq foot	70.7262
Kilograms	kg	Drams (apoth. or troy)	257.20597
		Drams (avdp.)	564.38339
		Grains	15,432.358
		Hundredweights (long)	0.019684131
		Hundredweights (short)	0.022046226
		Ounces (apoth. or troy)	32.150737
		Ounces (avdp.)	35.273962
		Pennyweights	643.01493
		Poundals	70.931635
		Pounds (apoth. or troy)	2.6792289
		Pounds (avdp.)	2.2046226
		Scruples (apoth.)	771.61792
		Tons (long)	0.00098420653
		Tons (metric)	0.001
		Tons (short)	0.0011023113
Kiloliters	kl	Cu centimeters	1×10^6
		Cu feet	35.31566
		Cu inches	61,025.45
		Cu meters	1.000028
		Cu yards	1.307987
		Gallons (Brit.)	219.9755
		Gallons (U. S., dry)	227.0271
		Gallons (U. S., liq.)	264.1794
		Liters	1000
Kilometers	km	Centimeters	100,000
		Feet	3280.8399
		Light years	1.05702×10^{-13}
		Meters	1000
		Miles (naut., int.)	0.53995680
		Miles (statute)	0.62137119
		Rods	198.83878
		Yards	1093.6133
Liters	l	Bushels (Brit.)	0.02749694
		Bushels (U. S.)	0.02837839
		Cu centimeters	1000
		Cu feet	0.03531566
		Cu inches	61.02545
		Cu meters	0.001
		Cu yards	0.001307987
		Drams (U. S., fluid)	270.5198
		Gallons (Brit.)	0.2199755
		Gallons (U. S., dry)	0.2270271
		Gallons (U. S., liq.)	0.2641794
		Gills (Brit.)	7.039217
		Gills (U. S.)	8.453742

To convert from unit	Abbreviation —symbol	To	Multiply by
Liters—cont'd		Minims (U. S.)	16,231.19
		Ounces (Brit., fluid)	35.19609
		Ounces (U. S., fluid)	33.81497
		Pecks (Brit.)	0.1099878
		Pecks (U. S.)	0.1135136
		Pints (Brit.)	1.759804
		Pints (U. S., dry)	1.816217
		Pints (U. S., liq.)	2.113436
		Quarts, (Brit.)	0.8799021
		Quarts (U. S., dry)	0.9081084
		Quarts (U. S., liq.)	1.056718
Meters	m	Ångström units	1×10^{10}
		Centimeters	100
		Feet	3.2808399
		Inches	39.370079
		Kilometers	0.001
		Megameters	1×10
		Miles (naut., Brit.)	0.00053961182
		Miles (naut., int.)	0.00053995680
		Miles (statute)	0.00062137119
		Millimeters	1000
		Nanometers	1×10^{9}
		Mils	39,370.079
		Rods	0.19883878
		Yards	1.0936133
Meters of Hg (0°C)		Atmospheres	1.3157895
		Feet of H_2O (60°F)	44.6474
		Inches of Hg (32°F)	39.370079
		Kilograms/sq centimeters	1.35951
		Pounds/sq inch	19.3368
Micrograms	μg	Grams	1×10^{-6}
		Milligrams	0.001
Micrometers	μm	Ångström units	10,000
		Centimeters	0.0001
		Feet	3.2808399×10^{-6}
		Inches	3.9370079×10^{-5}
		Meters	1×10^{-6}
		Millimeters	0.001
		Nanometers	1000
Miles (naut., Brit.)		Cable lengths	8.4390493
		Fathoms	1012.6859
		Feet	6076.1155
		Kilometers	1.852
		Meters	1852
		Miles (geographical)	1
		Miles (naut., Brit.)	0.99936110
		Miles (statute)	1.1507794
Miles (statute)		Centimeters	160,934.4
		Feet	5280
		Inches	63,360
		Kilometers	1.609344

To convert from unit	Abbreviation —symbol	To	Multiply by
Miles (statute)—cont'd		Meters	1609.344
		Miles (naut., Brit.)	0.86842105
		Miles (naut., int.)	0.86897624
		Rods	320
		Yards	1760
Milligrams	mg	Carats (1877)	0.004871
		Carats (metric)	0.005
		Drams (apoth. or troy)	0.00025720597
		Drams (advp.)	0.00056438339
Milliliters	ml	Cu centimeters	1
		Cu inches	0.06102545
		Drams (U. S., fluid)	0.2705198
		Gills (U. S.)	0.008453742
		Liters	0.001
		Minims (U. S.)	16.23119
		Ounces (Brit., fluid)	0.03519609
		Ounces (U. S., fluid)	0.3381497
		Pints (Brit.)	0.001759804
		Pints (U. S., liq.)	0.002113436
Millimeters	mm	Ångström units	1×10^7
		Centimeters	0.1
		Decimeters	0.01
		Dekameters	0.001
		Feet	0.0032808399
		Inches	0.039370079
		Meters	0.001
		Micrometers	1000
		Mils	39.370079
Millimeters of HG (0°C)	mm	Atmospheres	0.0013157895
		Bars	0.00133322
		Dynes/sq centimeter	1333.224
		Grams/sq centimeter	1.35951
		Kilograms/sq meter	13.5951
		Pounds/sq foot	2.78450
		Pounds/sq inch	0.0193368
		Torrs	1
Minims (Brit.)	min ℳ	Cu centimeter	0.05919385
		Cu inches	0.003612230
		Milliliters	0.05919219
		Ounces (Brit., fluid)	0.0020833333
		Scruples (Brit., fluid)	0.05
Minims (U. S.)	min ℳ	Cu centimeters	0.061611520
		Cu inches	0.0037597656
		Drams (U. S., fluid)	0.0166666
		Gallons (U. S., liq.)	1.6276042×10^{-5}
		Gills (U. S.)	0.0005208333
		Liters	6.160979×10^{-5}
		Milliliters	0.06160979
		Ounces (U. S., fluid)	0.002083333
		Pints (U. S., liq.)	0.0001302083

To convert from unit	Abbreviation —symbol	To	Multiply by
Nanometer	nm	Ångström Units	10
		Centimeters	1×10^{-7}
		Inches	3.9370079×10^{-8}
		Micrometers	0.001
		Millimeters	1×10^{-6}
Ounces (apoth. or troy)	oz ℥	Dekagrams	1.7554286
		Drams (apoth. or troy)	8
		Drams (avdp.)	17.554286
		Grains	480
		Grams	31.103486
		Milligrams	31,103.486
		Ounces (avdp.)	1.0971429
		Pennyweights	20
		Pounds (apoth. or troy)	0.0833333
		Pounds (avdp.)	0.068571429
		Scruples (apoth.)	24
Ounces (avdp.)	oz	Drams (apoth. or troy)	7.291666
		Drams (avdp.)	16
		Grains	437.5
		Grams	28.349523
		Hundredweights (long)	0.00055803571
		Hundredweights (short)	0.000625
		Ounces (apoth. or troy)	0.9114583
		Pennyweights	18.229166
		Pounds (apoth. or troy)	0.075954861
		Pounds (avdp.)	0.0625
		Scruples (apoth.)	21.875
Ounces (Brit., fluid)	oz	Cu centimeters	28.41305
		Cu inches	1.733870
		Drachms (Brit., fluid)	8
		Drams (U. S., fluid)	7.686075
		Gallons (Brit.)	0.00625
		Milliliters	28.41225
		Minims (Brit.)	480
		Ounces (U. S., fluid)	0.9607594
Ounces (U. S., fluid)	oz	Cu centimeters	29.573730
		Cu inches	1.8046875
		Cu meters	2.9573730×10^{-5}
		Drams (U. S., fluid)	8
		Gallons (U. S., dry)	0.0067138047
		Gallons (U. S., liq.)	0.0078125
		Gills (U. S.)	0.25
		Liters	0.029572702
		Minims (U. S.)	480
		Ounces (Brit., fluid)	1.040843
		Pints (U.S., liq.)	0.0625
		Quarts (U. S., liq.)	0.03125
Parts per million*	ppm	Grains/gallon (Brit.)	0.07015488
		Grains/gallon (U. S.)	0.058411620

*Based on density of 1 gram/ml for the solvent.

To convert from units	Abbreviation —symbol	To	Multiply by
Parts per million—cont'd		Grams/liter	0.001
		Milligrams/liter	1
Pecks (Brit.)	pk	Bushels (Brit.)	0.25
		Coombs (Brit.)	0.0625
		Cu centimeter	9092.175
		Cu inches	554.8385
		Gallons (Brit.)	2
		Gills (Brit.)	64
		Liters	9.091920
		Pints (Brit.)	16
		Quarts (Brit.)	8
		Quarts (U. S., dry)	8.256449
Pecks (U. S.)	pk	Barrels (U. S., dry)	0.076191185
		Bushels (U. S.)	0.25
		Cu centimeters	8809.7675
		Cu feet	0.311114005
		Cu inches	537.605
		Gallons (U. S., dry)	2
		Gallons (U. S., liq.)	2.3272944
		Liters	8.809521
		Pints (U. S., dry)	16
		Quarts (U. S., dry)	8
Pennyweights	dwt	Drams (apoth. or troy)	0.4
		Drams (avdp.)	0.87771429
		Grains	24
		Grams	1.55517384
		Ounces (apoth. or troy)	0.05
		Ounces (avdp.)	0.054857143
		Pounds (apoth. or troy)	0.0041666
		Pounds (avdp.)	0.0034285714
Pints (Brit.)	pt	Cu centimeter	568.26092
		Gallons (Brit.)	0.125
		Gills (Brit.)	4
		Gills (U. S.)	4.803797
		Liters	0.5682450
		Minims (Brit.)	9600
		Ounces (Brit., fluid)	20
		Pints (U. S., dry)	1.032056
		Pints (U. S., Liq.)	1.200949
		Quarts (Brit.)	0.5
		Scruples (Brit., fluid)	480
Pints (U. S., dry)	pt	Bushels (U. S.)	0.015625
		Cu centimeters	550.61047
		Cu inches	33.6003125
		Gallons (U. S., dry)	0.125
		Gallons (U. S., liq.)	0.14545590
		Liters	0.5505951
		Pecks (U. S.)	0.0625
		Quarts (U. S., dry)	0.5

To convert from unit	Abbreviation —symbol	To	Multiply by
Pints (U. S., liq.)	pt	Cu centimeters	473.17647
		Cu feet	0.016710069
		Cu inches	28.875
		Cu yards	0.00061889146
		Drams (U. S., fluid)	128
		Gallons (U. S., liq.)	0.125
		Gills (U. S.)	4
		Liters	0.4731632
		Milliliters	473.1632
		Minims (U. S.)	7680
		Ounces (U. S., fluid)	16
		Pints (Brit.)	0.8326747
		Quarts (U. S., liq.)	0.5
Poundals		Dynes	13,825.50
		Grams	14.09808
		Pounds (avdp.)	0.0310810
Pounds (apoth. or troy)	lb ap	Drams (apoth. or troy)	96
		Drams (avdp.)	210.65143
		Grains	5760
		Grams	373.24172
		Kilograms	0.37324172
		Ounces (apoth. or troy)	12
		Ounces (avdp.)	13.165714
		Pennyweights	240
		Pounds (avdp.)	0.8228571
		Scruples (apoth.)	288
		Tons (long)	0.00036734694
		Tons (metric)	0.00037324172
		Tons (short)	0.00041142857
Pounds (avdp.)	lb avdp.	Drams (apoth. or troy)	116.6666
		Drams (avdp.)	256
		Grains	7000
		Grams	453.59237
		Kilograms	0.45359237
		Ounces (apoth. or troy)	14.583333
		Ounces (avdp.)	16
		Pennyweights	291.6666
		Poundals	32.1740
		Pounds (apoth. or troy)	1.215277
		Scruples (apoth.)	350
		Slugs	0.0310810
		Tons (long)	0.00044642857
		Tons (metric)	0.00045359237
		Tons (short)	0.0005
Quarts (Brit.)	qt	Cu centimeters	1136.522
		Cu inches	69.35482
		Gallons (Brit.)	0.25
		Gallons (U. S., liq.)	0.3002373
		Liters	1.136490
		Quarts (U. S., dry)	1.032056
		Quarts (U. S., liq.)	1.200949

To convert from unit	Abbreviation —symbol	To	Multiply by
Quarts (U. S., dry)	qt	Bushels (U. S.)	0.03125
		Cu centimeters	1101.2209
		Cu feet	0.038889251
		Cu inches	67.200625
		Gallons (U. S., dry)	0.25
		Gallons (U. S., liq.)	0.29091180
		Liters	1.1011901
		Pecks (U. S.)	0.125
		Pints (U. S., dry)	2
Quarts (U. S., liq.)	qt	Cu centimeters	946.35295
		Cu feet	0.033420136
		Cu inches	57.75
		Drams (U. S., fluid)	256
		Gallons (U. S., dry)	0.21484175
		Gallons (U. S., liq.)	0.25
		Gills (U. S.)	8
		Liters	0.9463264
		Ounces (U. S., fluid)	32
		Pints (U. S., liq.)	2
		Quarts (Brit.)	0.8326747
		Quarts (U. S., dry)	0.8593670
Quintals (metric)		Grams	100,000
		Hundredweights (long)	1.9684131
		Kilograms	100
		Pounds (avdp.)	220.46226
Rods	rd	Centimeters	502.92
		Chains (Gunter's)	0.25
		Chains (Ramden's)	0.165
		Feet	16.5
		Furlongs	0.025
		Inches	198
		Links (Gunter's)	25
		Links (Ramden's)	16.5
		Meters	5.0292
		Miles (statute)	0.003125
		Yards	5.5
Rods (Brit., volume)	rd	Cu feet	1000
		Cu meters	28.316847
Scruples (apoth.)	s apoth	Drams (apoth. or troy)	0.333333
		Drams (avdp.)	0.73142857
		Grains	20
		Grams	1.2959782
		Ounces (apoth. or troy)	0.041666
		Ounces (avdp.)	0.045714286
		Pennyweights	0.833333
		Pounds (apoth. or troy)	0.003472222
		Pounds (avdp.)	0.0028571429
Scruples (Brit., fluid)		Minims (Brit.)	20

To convert from unit	Abbreviation —symbol	To	Multiply by
Square feet	ft^2	Acres	2.295684×10^{-5}
		Ares	0.0009290304
		Sq centimeters	929.0304
		Sq inches	144
		Sq meters	0.09290304
		Sq miles	3.5870064×10^{-8}
		Sq rods	0.0036730946
		Sq yards	0.111111
Square inches	in^2	Circular mils	1,273,239.5
		Sq centimeters	6.4516
		Sq decimeters	0.064516
		Sq feet	0.0069444
		Sq meters	0.00064516
		Sq miles	$2.4909767 \times 10^{-10}$
		Sq mm	645.16
		Sq mils	1×10^6
Square kilometers	km^2	Acres	247.10538
		Sq feet	1.0763910×10^7
		Sq inches	1.5500031×10^9
		Sq meters	1×10^6
		Sq miles	0.38610216
Square meters	m^2	Acres	0.00024710538
		Ares	0.01
		Hectares	0.0001
		Sq centimeters	10,000
		Sq feet	10.763910
		Sq inches	1550.0031
		Sq kilometers	1×10^{-6}
		Sq miles	3.8610216×10^{-7}
		Sq rods	0.039536861
Square miles	mi^2	Acres	640
		Hectares	258.99881
		Sq feet	2.7878288×10^7
		Sq kilometers	2.5899881
		Sq meters	2589988.1
		Sq rods	102,400
		Sq yards	3.0976×10^6
Square millimeters	mm^2	Sq centimeters	0.01
		Sq inches	0.0015500031
		Sq meters	1×10^{-6}
Square rods	rd^2	Acres	0.00625
		Ares	0.2529285264
		Hectares	0.002529285264
		Sq centimeters	252,928.5264
		Sq feet	272.25
		Sq feet (U. S. survey)	272.24891
		Sq inches	39,204
		Sq meters	25.29285264
		Sq miles	9.765625×10^{-6}
		Sq yards	30.25

To convert from unit	Abbreviation —symbol	To	Multiply by
Square yards	yd^2	Acres	0.00020661157
		Ares	0.0083612736
		Hectares	8.3612736×10^{-5}
		Sq centimeters	8361.2736
		Sq feet	9
		Sq feet (U. S. survey)	8.9999640
		Sq inches	1296
		Sq meters	0.83612736
		Sq miles	$3.228305785 \times 10^{-7}$
		Sq rods	0.033057851
Tons (long)	t	Kilograms	1016.0469
		Ounces (avdp.)	35,840
		Pounds (apoth. or troy)	2722.22
		Pounds (avdp.)	2240
		Tons (metric)	1.0160469
		Tons (short)	1.12
Tons (metric)	t	Grams	1×10^6
		Hundredweights (short)	22.046226
		Kilograms	1000
		Ounces (avdp.)	35,273.962
		Pounds (apoth. or troy)	2679.2289
		Pounds (avdp.)	2204.6226
		Tons (long)	0.98420653
		Tons (short)	1.1023113
Tons (short)	t	Hundredweights (short)	20
		Kilograms	907.18474
		Ounces (avdp.)	32,000
		Pounds (apoth. or troy)	2430.555
		Pounds (avdp.)	2000
		Tons (long)	0.89285714
		Tons (metric)	0.90718474
Yards	yd	Centimeters	91.44
		Chains (Gunter's)	0.454545454
		Chains (Ramden's)	0.03
		Cubits	2
		Fathoms	0.5
		Feet	3
		Feet (U. S. survey)	2.9999940
		Furlongs	0.00454545
		Inches	36
		Meters	0.9144
		Quarters (Brit., linear)	4
		Rods	0.181818
Years (calendar)	yr	Days (mean solar)	365
		Hours (mean solar)	8760
		Minutes (mean solar)	525,600
		Months (lunar)	12.360065
		Months (mean calendar)	12
		Seconds (mean solar)	3.1536×10^7
		Weeks (mean calendar)	52.142857
		Years (sidereal)	0.99929814
		Years (tropical)	0.99933690

Conversion factors for the more common electrolytes

Electrolyte	Unit reported in	×	Factor	=	Desired unit
Ca	mg/dl		0.5		mEq/l
Ca	mEq/l		2.0		mg/dl
Cl	mg/dl		0.282		mEq/l (as Cl)
Cl	mg/dl		0.282		mEq/l (as NaCl)
Cl	mEq/l		3.55		mg/dl (as Cl)
Cl	mEq/l		5.85		mg/dl (as NaCl)
Cl	mEq/l		0.0585		gm/l (as NaCl)
CO_2	vol%		0.45		mEq/l
CO_2	mEq/l		2.226		vol%
K	mg/dl		0.256		mEq/l
K	mEq/l		3.91		mg/dl
K	mEq/l		0.0746		gm/l (as KCl)
Na	mg/dl		0.435		mEq/l (as Na)
Na	mg/dl		0.435		mEq/l (as NaCl)
Na	mEq/l		2.3		mg/dl (as Na)
Na	mEq/l		5.85		mg/dl (as NaCl)
Na	mEq/l		0.0585		gm/l (as NaCl)

Conversion factors for converting conventional enzyme units to international units per liter (mU/ml)

Enzyme	One conventional unit	=	IU/l
Acid phosphatase			
Bodansky	37°C, 1 mg P/hr/100 ml		5.37
Shinowara-Jones-Reinhart			5.37
King-Armstrong	37°C, 1 mg phenol/hr/100 ml		1.77
Kind-King			1.77
Bessey-Lowry-Brock	37°C, 1 mmole p-nitrophenol/hr/1000 ml		16.67
Gutman-Gutman			1.77
Aldolase			
Sibley-Lehninger	1 μl(0.0446 μmole) fructose, 1,6-diphosphate/ hr/ml		0.74
Burns	37°C, 1 μl fructose 1,6-diphosphate/hr/ml		0.61
Schapira et al.	37°C, 1 mg triosephosphate-p/min/1000 ml		16.0
Alkaline phosphatase			
Bodansky	37°C, 1 mg P/hr/100 ml		5.37
Shinowara-Jones-Reinhart	37°C, 1 mg P/hr/100 ml		5.37
King-Armstrong	37°C, 1 mg phenol/15 min/100 ml		7.1
Kind-King	1 mg phenol/15 min/100 ml		7.06
Bessey-Lowry-Brock	37°C, 1 mmole p-nitrophenol/hr/1000 ml		16.67
Babson	1 μmole phenolphthalein/min/1000 ml		1.0
Bowers-McComb	1 μmole p-nitrophenol/min/1000 ml		1.0
Amylase			
Somogyi (saccharogenic)	40°C, 1 mg glucose/30 min/100 ml		1.85
Somogyi	37°C, 5 mg starch/15 min/100 ml		20.6
Cholinesterase			
de la Huerga	37°C, 1 μmole acetylcholine/hr/ml		16.7
Hydroxybutyric dehydrogenase			
Rosalki-Wilkinson	ΔA_{340} 0.001/min/ml (V_t, 3 ml) (NADH)		0.482
Isocitrate dehydrogenase			
Wolfson-Williams-Ashman	25°C, 1 nmole NADH/hr/ml		0.0167
Taylor-Friedman			0.0167
Lactate dehydrogenase			
Wroblewski-LaDue	ΔA_{340} 0.001/min/ml (V_t, 3 ml) (NADH)		0.482
Wroblewski-Gregory			0.482
Lipase			
Cherry-Crandall (Tietz-Fiereck)	50 μmoles of fatty acid/3 hr/ml		277
Malic dehydrogenase			
Wacker-Ulmer-Valee			0.482
Transaminase			
Reitman-Frankel			0.482
Karmen	25°C ΔA_{340} 0.001/min/ml (V_t, 3 ml) (NADH)		0.482

Temperature conversion table

To Convert			To Convert			To Convert		
To °C	←°F or °C→	To °F	To °C	←°F or °C→	To °F	To °C	←°F or °C→	To °F
−190	−310	—	−156.67	−250	−418	−123.33	−190	−310
−189.44	−309	—	−156.11	−249	−416.2	−122.78	−189	−308.2
−188.89	−308	—	−155.56	−248	−414.4	−122.22	−188	−306.4
−188.33	−307	—	−155	−247	−412.6	−121.67	−187	−304.6
−187.78	−306	—	−154.44	−246	−410.8	−121.11	−186	−302.8
−187.22	−305	—	−153.89	−245	−409	−120.56	−185	−301
−186.67	−304	—	−153.33	−244	−407.2	−120	−184	−299.2
−186.11	−303	—	−152.78	−243	−405.4	−119.44	−183	−297.4
−185.56	−302	—	−152.22	−242	−403.6	−118.89	−182	−295.6
−185	−301	—	−151.67	−241	−401.8	−118.33	−181	−293.8
−184.44	−300	—	−151.11	−240	−400	−117.78	−180	−292
−183.89	−299	—	−150.56	−239	−398.2	−117.22	−179	−290.2
−183.33	−298	—	−150	−238	−396.4	−116.67	−178	−288.4
−182.78	−297	—	−149.44	−237	−394.6	−116.11	−177	−286.6
−182.22	−296	—	−148.89	−236	−392.8	−115.56	−176	−284.8
−181.67	−295	—	−148.33	−235	−391	−115	−175	−283
−181.11	−294	—	−147.78	−234	−389.2	−114.44	−174	−281.2
−180.56	−293	—	−147.22	−233	−387.4	−113.89	−173	−279.4
−180	−292	—	−146.67	−232	−385.6	−113.33	−172	−277.6
−179.44	−291	—	−146.11	−231	−383.8	−112.78	−171	−275.8
−178.89	−290	—	−145.56	−230	−382	−112.22	−170	−274
−178.33	−289	—	−145	−229	−380.2	−111.67	−169	−272.2
−177.78	−288	—	−144.44	−228	−378.4	−111.11	−168	−270.4
−177.22	−287	—	−143.89	−227	−376.6	−110.56	−167	−268.6
−176.67	−286	—	−143.33	−226	−374.8	−110	−166	−266.8
−176.11	−285	—	−142.78	−225	−373	−109.44	−165	−265
−175.56	−284	—	−142.22	−224	−371.2	−108.89	−164	−263.2
−175	−283	—	−141.67	−223	−369.4	−108.33	−163	−261.4
−174.44	−282	—	−141.11	−222	−367.6	−107.78	−162	−259.6
−173.89	−281	—	−140.56	−221	−365.8	−107.22	−161	−257.8
−173.33	−280	—	−140	−220	−364	−106.67	−160	−256
−172.78	−279	—	−139.44	−219	−362.2	−106.11	−159	−254.2
−172.22	−278	—	−138.89	−218	−360.4	−105.56	−158	−252.4
−171.67	−277	—	−138.33	−217	−358.6	−105	−157	−250.6
−171.11	−276	—	−137.78	−216	−356.8	−104.44	−156	−248.8
−170.56	−275	—						
−170	−274	—	−137.22	−215	−355	−103.89	−155	−247
—	−273.15	−459.67	−136.67	−214	−353.2	−103.33	−154	−245.2
−169.44	−273	−459.4	−136.11	−213	−351.4	−102.78	−153	−243.4
−168.89	−272	−457.6	−135.56	−212	−349.6	−102.22	−152	−241.6
−168.33	−271	−455.8	−135	−211	−347.8	−101.67	−151	−239.8
−167.78	−270	−454	−134.44	−210	−346	−101.11	−150	−238
−167.22	−269	−452.2	−133.89	−209	−344.2	−100.56	−149	−236.2
−166.67	−268	−450.4	−133.33	−208	−342.4	−100	−148	−234.4
−166.11	−267	−448.6	−132.78	−207	−340.6	−99.44	−147	−232.6
−165.56	−266	−446.8	−132.22	−206	−338.8	−98.89	−146	−230.8
−165	−265	−445	−131.67	−205	−337	−98.33	−145	−229
−164.44	−264	−443.2	−131.11	−204	−335.2	−97.78	−144	−227.2
−163.89	−263	−441.4	−130.56	−203	−333.4	−97.22	−143	−225.4
−163.33	−262	−439.6	−130	−202	−331.6	−96.67	−142	−223.6
−162.78	−261	−437.8	−129.44	−201	−329.8	−96.11	−141	−221.8
−162.22	−260	−436	−128.89	−200	−328	−95.56	−140	−220
−161.67	−259	−434.2	−128.33	−199	−326.2	−95	−139	−218.2
−161.11	−258	−432.4	−127.78	−198	−324.4	−94.44	−138	−216.4
−160.56	−257	−430.6	−127.22	−197	−322.6	−93.89	−137	−214.6
−160	−256	−428.8	−126.67	−196	−320.8	−93.33	−136	−212.8
−159.44	−255	−427	−126.11	−195	−319	−92.78	−135	−211
−158.89	−254	−425.2	−125.56	−194	−317.2	−92.22	−134	−209.2
−158.33	−253	−423.4	−125	−193	−315.4	−91.67	−133	−207.4
−157.78	−252	−421.6	−124.44	−192	−313.6	−91.11	−132	−205.6
−157.22	−251	−419.8	−123.89	−191	−311.8	−90.56	−131	−203.8

From Handbook of chemistry and physics, ed. 50, Weast, R. C., editor, 1969. Used by permission of CRC Press, Inc.

To Convert			To Convert			To Convert		
To °C	←°F or °C→	To °F	To °C	←°F or °C→	To °F	To °C	←°F or °C→	To °F
−90	−130	−202	−56.67	−70	−94	−23.33	−10	14
−89.44	−129	−200.2	−56.11	−69	−92.2	−22.78	−9	15.8
−88.89	−128	−198.4	−55.56	−68	−90.4	−22.22	−8	17.6
−88.33	−127	−196.6	−55	−67	−88.6	−21.67	−7	19.4
−87.78	−126	−194.8	−54.44	−66	−86.8	−21.11	−6	21.2
−87.22	−125	−193	−53.89	−65	−85	−20.56	−5	23
−86.67	−124	−191.2	−53.33	−64	−83.2	−20	−4	24.8
−86.11	−123	−189.4	−52.78	−63	−81.4	−19.44	−3	26.6
−85.56	−122	−187.6	−52.22	−62	−79.6	−18.89	−2	28.4
−85	−121	−185.8	−51.67	−61	−77.8	−18.33	−1	30.2
−84.44	−120	−184	−51.11	−60	−76	−17.78	0	32
−83.89	−119	−182.2	−50.56	−59	−74.2	−17.22	1	33.8
−83.33	−118	−180.4	−50	−58	−72.4	−16.67	2	35.6
−82.78	−117	−178.6	−49.44	−57	−70.6	−16.11	3	37.4
−82.22	−116	−176.8	−48.89	−56	−68.8	−15.56	4	39.2
−81.67	−115	−175	−48.33	−55	−67	−15	5	41
−81.11	−114	−173.2	−47.78	−54	−65.2	−14.44	6	42.8
−80.56	−113	−171.4	−47.22	−53	−63.4	−13.89	7	44.6
−80	−112	−169.6	−46.67	−52	−61.6	−13.33	8	46.4
−79.44	−111	−167.8	−46.11	−51	−59.8	−12.78	9	48.2
−78.89	−110	−166	−45.56	−50	−58	−12.22	10	50
−78.33	−109	−164.2	−45	−49	−56.2	−11.67	11	51.8
−77.78	−108	−162.4	−44.44	−48	−54.4	−11.11	12	53.6
−77.22	−107	−160.6	−43.89	−47	−52.6	−10.56	13	55.4
−76.67	−106	−158.8	−43.33	−46	−50.8	−10	14	57.2
−76.11	−105	−157	−42.78	−45	−49	−9.44	15	59
−75.56	−104	−155.2	−42.22	−44	−47.2	−8.89	16	60.8
−75	−103	−153.4	−41.67	−43	−45.4	−8.33	17	62.6
−74.44	−102	−151.6	−41.11	−42	−43.6	−7.78	18	64.4
−73.89	−101	−149.8	−40.56	−41	−41.8	−7.22	19	66.2
−73.33	−100	−148	−40	−40	−40	−6.67	20	68
−72.78	−99	−146.2	−39.44	−39	−38.2	−6.11	21	69.8
−72.22	−98	−144.4	−38.89	−38	−36.4	−5.56	22	71.6
−71.67	−97	−142.6	−38.33	−37	−34.6	−5	23	73.4
−71.11	−96	−140.8	−37.78	−36	−32.8	−4.44	24	75.2
−70.56	−95	−139	−37.22	−35	−31	−3.89	25	77
−70	−94	−137.2	−36.67	−34	−29.2	−3.33	26	78.8
−69.44	−93	−135.4	−36.11	−33	−27.4	−2.78	27	80.6
−68.89	−92	−133.6	−35.56	−32	−25.6	−2.22	28	82.4
−68.33	−91	−131.8	−35	−31	−23.8	−1.67	29	84.2
−67.78	−90	−130	−34.44	−30	−22	−1.11	30	86
−67.22	−89	−128.2	−33.89	−29	−20.2	−0.56	31	87.8
−66.67	−88	−126.4	−33.33	−28	−18.4	0	32	89.6
−66.11	−87	−124.6	−32.78	−27	−16.6	.56	33	91.4
−65.56	−86	−122.8	−32.22	−26	−14.8	1.11	34	93.2
−65	−85	−121	−31.67	−25	−13	1.67	35	95
−64.44	−84	−119.2	−31.11	−24	−11.2	2.22	36	96.8
−63.89	−83	−117.4	−30.56	−23	−9.4	2.78	37	98.6
−63.33	−82	−115.6	−30	−22	−7.6	3.33	38	100.4
−62.78	−81	−113.8	−29.44	−21	−5.8	3.89	39	102.2
−62.22	−80	−112	−28.89	−20	−4	4.44	40	104
−61.67	−79	−110.2	−28.33	−19	−2.2	5	41	105.8
−61.11	−78	−108.4	−27.78	−18	−0.4	5.56	42	107.6
−60.56	−77	−106.6	−27.22	−17	1.4	6.11	43	109.4
−60	−76	−104.8	−26.67	−16	3.2	6.67	44	111.2
−59.44	−75	−103	−26.11	−15	5	7.22	45	113
−58.89	−74	−101.2	−25.56	−14	6.8	7.78	46	114.8
−58.33	−73	−99.4	−25	−13	8.6	8.33	47	116.6
−57.78	−72	−97.6	−24.44	−12	10.4	8.89	48	118.4
−57.22	−71	−95.8	−23.89	−11	12.2	9.44	49	120.2

To °C	←°F or °C→	To °F	To °C	←°F or °C→	To °F	To °C	←°F or °C→	To °F
10	**50**	122	43.33	**110**	230	76.67	**170**	338
10.56	**51**	123.8	43.89	**111**	231.8	77.22	**171**	339.8
11.11	**52**	125.6	44.44	**112**	233.6	77.78	**172**	341.6
11.67	**53**	127.4	45	**113**	235.4	78.33	**173**	343.4
12.22	**54**	129.2	45.56	**114**	237.2	78.89	**174**	345.2
12.78	**55**	131	46.11	**115**	239	79.44	**175**	347
13.33	**56**	132.8	46.67	**116**	240.8	80	**176**	348.8
13.89	**57**	134.6	47.22	**117**	242.6	80.56	**177**	350.6
14.44	**58**	136.4	47.78	**118**	244.4	81.11	**178**	352.4
15	**59**	138.2	48.33	**119**	246.2	81.67	**179**	354.2
15.56	**60**	140	48.89	**120**	248	82.22	**180**	356
16.11	**61**	141.8	49.44	**121**	249.8	82.78	**181**	357.8
16.67	**62**	143.6	50	**122**	251.6	83.33	**182**	359.6
17.22	**63**	145.4	50.56	**123**	253.4	83.89	**183**	361.4
17.78	**64**	147.2	51.11	**124**	255.2	84.44	**184**	363.2
18.33	**65**	149	51.67	**125**	257	85	**185**	365
18.89	**66**	150.8	52.22	**126**	258.8	85.56	**186**	366.8
19.44	**67**	152.6	52.78	**127**	260.6	86.11	**187**	368.6
20	**68**	154.4	53.33	**128**	262.4	86.67	**188**	370.4
20.56	**69**	156.2	53.89	**129**	264.2	87.22	**189**	372.2
21.11	**70**	158	54.44	**130**	266	87.78	**190**	374
21.67	**71**	159.8	55	**131**	267.8	88.33	**191**	375.8
22.22	**72**	161.6	55.56	**132**	269.6	88.89	**192**	377.6
22.78	**73**	163.4	56.11	**133**	271.4	89.44	**193**	379.4
23.33	**74**	165.2	56.67	**134**	273.2	90	**194**	381.2
23.89	**75**	167	57.22	**135**	275	90.56	**195**	383
24.44	**76**	168.8	57.78	**136**	276.8	91.11	**196**	384.8
25	**77**	170.6	58.33	**137**	278.6	91.67	**197**	386.6
25.56	**78**	172.4	58.89	**138**	280.4	92.22	**198**	388.4
26.11	**79**	174.2	59.44	**139**	282.2	92.78	**199**	390.2
26.67	**80**	176	60	**140**	284	93.33	**200**	392
27.22	**81**	177.8	60.56	**141**	285.8	93.89	**201**	393.8
27.78	**82**	179.6	61.11	**142**	287.6	94.44	**202**	395.6
28.33	**83**	181.4	61.67	**143**	289.4	95	**203**	397.4
28.89	**84**	183.2	62.22	**144**	291.2	95.56	**204**	399.2
29.44	**85**	185	62.78	**145**	293	96.11	**205**	401
30	**86**	186.8	63.33	**146**	294.8	96.67	**206**	402.8
30.56	**87**	188.6	63.89	**147**	296.6	97.22	**207**	404.6
31.11	**88**	190.4	64.44	**148**	298.4	97.78	**208**	406.4
31.67	**89**	192.2	65	**149**	300.2	98.33	**209**	408.2
32.22	**90**	194	65.56	**150**	302	98.89	**210**	410
32.78	**91**	195.8	66.11	**151**	303.8	99.44	**211**	411.8
33.33	**92**	197.6	66.67	**152**	305.6	100	**212**	413.6
33.89	**93**	199.4	67.22	**153**	307.4	100.56	**213**	415.4
34.44	**94**	201.2	67.78	**154**	309.2	101.11	**214**	417.2
35	**95**	203	68.33	**155**	311	101.67	**215**	419
35.56	**96**	204.8	68.89	**156**	312.8	102.22	**216**	420.8
36.11	**97**	206.6	69.44	**157**	314.6	102.78	**217**	422.6
36.67	**98**	208.4	70	**158**	316.4	103.33	**218**	424.4
37.22	**99**	210.2	70.56	**159**	318.2	103.89	**219**	426.2
37.78	**100**	212	71.11	**160**	320	104.44	**220**	428
38.33	**101**	213.8	71.67	**161**	321.8	105	**221**	429.8
38.89	**102**	215.6	72.22	**162**	323.6	105.56	**222**	431.6
39.44	**103**	217.4	72.78	**163**	325.4	106.11	**223**	433.4
40	**104**	219.2	73.33	**164**	327.2	106.67	**224**	435.2
40.56	**105**	221	73.89	**165**	329	107.22	**225**	437
41.11	**106**	222.8	74.44	**166**	330.8	107.78	**226**	438.8
41.67	**107**	224.6	75	**167**	332.6	108.33	**227**	440.6
42.22	**108**	226.4	75.56	**168**	334.4	108.89	**228**	442.4
42.78	**109**	228.2	76.11	**169**	336.2	109.44	**229**	444.2

To Convert			To Convert			To Convert		
To °C	←°F or °C→	To °F	To °C	←°F or °C→	To °F	To °C	←°F or °C→	To °F
110	**230**	446	143.33	**290**	554	176.67	**350**	662
110.56	**231**	447.8	143.89	**291**	555.8	177.22	**351**	663.8
111.11	**232**	449.6	144.44	**292**	557.6	177.78	**352**	665.6
111.67	**233**	451.4	145	**293**	559.4	178.33	**353**	667.4
112.22	**234**	453.2	145.56	**294**	561.2	178.89	**354**	669.2
112.78	**235**	455	146.11	**295**	563	179.44	**355**	671
113.33	**236**	456.8	146.67	**296**	564.8	180	**356**	672.8
113.89	**237**	458.6	147.22	**297**	566.6	180.56	**357**	674.6
114.44	**238**	460.4	147.78	**298**	568.4	181.11	**358**	676.4
115	**239**	462.2	148.33	**299**	570.2	181.67	**359**	678.2
115.56	**240**	464	148.89	**300**	572	182.22	**360**	680
116.11	**241**	465.8	149.44	**301**	573.8	182.78	**361**	681.8
116.67	**242**	467.6	150	**302**	575.6	183.33	**362**	683.6
117.22	**243**	469.4	150.56	**303**	577.4	183.89	**363**	685.4
117.78	**244**	471.2	151.11	**304**	579.2	184.44	**364**	687.2
118.33	**245**	473	151.67	**305**	581	185	**365**	689
118.89	**246**	474.8	152.22	**306**	582.8	185.56	**366**	690.8
119.44	**247**	476.6	152.78	**307**	584.6	186.11	**367**	692.6
120	**248**	478.4	153.33	**308**	586.4	186.67	**368**	694.4
120.56	**249**	480.2	153.89	**309**	588.2	187.22	**369**	696.2
121.11	**250**	482	154.44	**310**	590	187.78	**370**	698
121.67	**251**	483.8	155	**311**	591.8	188.33	**371**	699.8
122.22	**252**	485.6	155.56	**312**	593.6	188.89	**372**	701.6
122.78	**253**	487.4	156.11	**313**	595.4	189.44	**373**	703.4
123.33	**254**	489.2	156.67	**314**	597.2	190	**374**	705.2
123.89	**255**	491	157.22	**315**	599	190.56	**375**	707
124.44	**256**	492.8	157.78	**316**	600.8	191.11	**376**	708.8
125	**257**	494.6	158.33	**317**	602.6	191.67	**377**	710.6
125.56	**258**	496.4	158.89	**318**	604.4	192.22	**378**	712.4
126.11	**259**	498.2	159.44	**319**	606.2	192.78	**379**	714.2
126.67	**260**	500	160	**320**	608	193.33	**380**	716
127.22	**261**	501.8	160.56	**321**	609.8	193.89	**381**	717.8
127.78	**262**	503.6	161.11	**322**	611.6	194.44	**382**	719.6
128.33	**263**	505.4	161.67	**323**	613.4	195	**383**	721.4
128.89	**264**	507.2	162.22	**324**	615.2	195.56	**384**	723.2
129.44	**265**	509	162.78	**325**	617	196.11	**385**	725
130	**266**	510.8	163.33	**326**	618.8	196.67	**386**	726.8
130.56	**267**	512.6	163.89	**327**	620.6	197.22	**387**	728.6
131.11	**268**	514.4	164.44	**328**	622.4	197.78	**388**	730.4
131.67	**269**	516.2	165	**329**	624.2	198.33	**389**	732.2
132.22	**270**	518	165.56	**330**	626	198.89	**390**	734
132.78	**271**	519.8	166.11	**331**	627.8	199.44	**391**	735.8
133.33	**272**	521.6	166.67	**332**	629.6	200	**392**	737.6
133.89	**273**	523.4	167.22	**333**	631.4	200.56	**393**	739.4
134.44	**274**	525.2	167.78	**334**	633.2	201.11	**394**	741.2
135	**275**	527	168.33	**335**	635	201.67	**395**	743
135.56	**276**	528.8	168.89	**336**	636.8	202.22	**396**	744.8
136.11	**277**	530.6	169.44	**337**	638.6	202.78	**397**	746.6
136.67	**278**	532.4	170	**338**	640.4	203.33	**398**	748.4
137.22	**279**	534.2	170.56	**339**	642.2	203.89	**399**	750.2
137.78	**280**	536	171.11	**340**	644	204.44	**400**	752
138.33	**281**	537.8	171.67	**341**	645.8	205	**401**	753.8
138.89	**282**	539.6	172.22	**342**	647.6	205.56	**402**	755.6
139.44	**283**	541.4	172.78	**343**	649.4	206.11	**403**	757.4
140	**284**	543.2	173.33	**344**	651.2	206.67	**404**	759.2
140.56	**285**	545	173.89	**345**	653	207.22	**405**	761
141.11	**286**	546.8	174.44	**346**	654.8	207.78	**406**	762.8
141.67	**287**	548.6	175	**347**	656.6	208.33	**407**	764.6
142.22	**288**	550.4	175.56	**348**	658.4	208.89	**408**	766.4
142.78	**289**	552.2	176.11	**349**	660.2	209.44	**409**	768.2

Periodic chart of the elements

NOBLE GASES

IA	IIA	IIIB	IVB	VB	VIB	VIIB	VIII	VIII	VIII	IB	IIB	IIIA	IVA	VA	VIA	VIIA	
1 H 1.0079†																	2 He 4.00260
3 Li 6.941†	4 Be 9.01218											5 B 10.81	6 C 12.011	7 N 14.0067	8 O 15.9994†	9 F 18.99840	10 Ne 20.179†
11 Na 22.98977	12 Mg 24.305											13 Al 26.98154	14 Si 28.086†	15 P 30.97376	16 S 32.06	17 Cl 35.453	18 Ar 39.948†
19 K 39.098†	20 Ca 40.08	21 Sc 44.9559	22 Ti 47.90†	23 V 50.9414†	24 Cr 51.996	25 Mn 54.9380	26 Fe 55.847†	27 Co 58.9332	28 Ni 58.70†	29 Cu 63.546†	30 Zn 65.38	31 Ga 69.72	32 Ge 72.59†	33 As 74.9216	34 Se 78.96†	35 Br 79.904	36 Kr 83.80
37 Rb 85.4678†	38 Sr 87.62	39 Y 88.9059	40 Zr 91.22	41 Nb 92.9064	42 Mo 95.94†	43 Tc 98.9062	44 Ru 101.07†	45 Rh 102.9055	46 Pd 106.4	47 Ag 107.868	48 Cd 112.40	49 In 114.82	50 Sn 118.69†	51 Sb 121.75†	52 Te 127.60†	53 I 126.9045	54 Xe 131.30
55 Cs 132.9054	56 Ba 137.34†	57 *La 138.9055†	72 Hf 178.49†	73 Ta 180.9479†	74 W 183.85†	75 Re 186.207	76 Os 190.2	77 Ir 192.22†	78 Pt 195.09†	79 Au 196.9665	80 Hg 200.59†	81 Tl 204.37†	82 Pb 207.2	83 Bi 208.9804	84 Po (210)	85 At (210)	86 Rn (222)
87 Fr (223)	88 Ra 226.0254	89 †Ac (227)	104 §(260)	105 §(260)													

*Lanthanoid Series

58 Ce 140.12	59 Pr 140.9077	60 Nd 144.24†	61 Pm (147)	62 Sm 150.4	63 Eu 151.96	64 Gd 157.25†	65 Tb 158.9254	66 Dy 162.50†	67 Ho 164.9304	68 Er 167.26†	69 Tm 168.9342	70 Yb 173.04†	71 Lu 174.97

†Actinoid Series

90 Th 232.0381	91 Pa 231.0359	92 U 238.029	93 Np 237.0482	94 Pu (244)	95 Am (243)	96 Cm (247)	97 Bk (247)	98 Cf (251)	99 Es (254)	100 Fm (257)	101 Md (258)	102 No (255)	103 Lr (256)

FISHER SCIENTIFIC COMPANY CAT. NO. 5-702-10

§The International Union for Pure and Applied Chemistry has not adopted official names or symbols for these elements.

†These weights are considered reliable to ±3 in the last place. Other weights are reliable to ±1 in the last place.

Atomic weights corrected to conform to the 1973 values of the Commission on Atomic Weights.

© Copyright 1973 Fisher Scientific Company

Used with permission of the Fisher Scientific Company, Pittsburgh, Pa.

Atomic weights

For the sake of completeness all known elements are included in the list. Several of those more recently discovered are represented only by the unstable isotopes. The value in parenthesis in the atomic weight column is, in each case, the mass number of the most stable isotope.**

Name	Symbol	At. No.	International atomic weight 1966	International atomic weight 1959	Valence
Actinium	Ac	89	....	(227)	....
Aluminum	Al	13	26.9815	26.98	3
Americium	Am	95	....	(243)	3, 4, 5, 6
Antimony, stibium	Sb	51	121.75	121.76	3, 5
Argon	Ar	18	39.948	39.944	0
Arsenic	As	33	74.9216	74.92	3, 5
Astatine	At	85	....	(210)	1, 3, 5, 7
Barium	Ba	56	137.34	137.36	2
Berkelium	Bk	97	....	(247)	3, 4
Beryllium	Be	4	9.0122	9.013	2
Bismuth	Bi	83	208.980	208.99	3, 5
Boron	B	5	10.811	10.82	3
Bromine	Br	35	79.904[1]	79.916	1, 3, 5, 7
Cadmium	Cd	48	112.40	112.41	2
Calcium	Ca	20	40.08	40.08	2
Californium	Cf	98	....	(251)	....
Carbon	C	6	12.01115	12.011	2, 4
Cerium	Ce	58	140.12	140.13	3, 4
Cesium	Cs	55	132.905	132.91	1
Chlorine	Cl	17	35.453	35.457	1, 3, 5, 7
Chromium	Cr	24	51.996	52.01	2, 3, 6
Cobalt	Co	27	58.9332	58.94	2, 3
Columbium, see *Niobium*					
Copper	Cu	29	63.546[2]	63.54	1, 2
Curium	Cm	96	....	(247)	3
Dysprosium	Dy	66	162.50	162.51	3
Einsteinium	Es	99	....	(254)	....
Erbium	Er	68	167.26	167.27	3
Europium	Eu	63	151.96	152.0	2, 3
Fermium	Fm	100	....	(257)	....
Fluorine	F	9	18.9984	19.00	1
Francium	Fr	87	....	(223)	1
Gadolinium	Gd	64	157.25	157.26	3
Gallium	Ga	31	69.72	69.72	2, 3
Germanium	Ge	32	72.59	72.60	4
Gold, aurum	Au	79	196.967	197.0	1, 3
Hafnium	Hf	72	178.49	178.50	4
Helium	He	2	4.0026	4.003	0
Holmium	Ho	67	164.930	164.94	3
Hydrogen	H	1	1.00797	1.0080	1
Indium	In	49	114.82	114.82	3
Iodine	I	53	126.9044	126.91	1, 3, 5 7
Iridium	Ir	77	192.2	192.2	3, 4
Iron, ferrum	Fe	26	55.847	55.85	2, 3
Krypton	Kr	36	83.80	83.80	0
Lanthanum	La	57	138.91	138.92	3
Lawrencium	Lr	103	(257)		
Lead, plumbum	Pb	82	207.19	207.21	2, 4
Lithium	Li	3	6.939	6.940	1
Lutetium	Lu	71	174.97	174.94	3
Magnesium	Mg	12	24.312	24.32	2
Manganese	Mn	25	54.9380	54.94	2, 3, 4, 6, 7
Mendelevium	Md	101	....	(256)	....
Mercury, hydrargyrum	Hg	80	200.59	200.61	1, 2
Molybdenum	Mo	42	95.94	95.95	3. 4. 6
Neodymium	Nd	60	144.24	144.27	3
Neon	Ne	10	20.183	20.183	0
Neptunium	Np	93	....	(237)	4, 5, 6
Nickel	Ni	28	58.71	58.71	2, 3
Niobium (columbium)	Nb	41	92.906	92.91	3, 5
Nitrogen	N	7	14.0067	14.008	3, 5
Nobelium	No	102	....	(254)	....
Osmium	Os	76	190.2	190.2	2, 3, 4, 8
Oxygen	O	8	15.9994	16.000	2
Palladium	Pd	46	106.4	106.4	2, 4, 6
Phosphorus	P	15	30.9738	30.975	3, 5
Platinum	Pt	78	195.09	195.09	2, 4
Plutonium	Pu	94	....	(244)	3, 4, 5, 6
Polonium	Po	84	....	(209)	....
Potassium, kalium	K	19	39.102	39.100	1
Praseodymium	Pr	59	140.907	140.92	3
Promethium	Pm	61	....	(145)	3
Protactinium	Pa	91	....	(231)	....
Radium	Ra	88	....	(226)	2
Radon	Rn	86	....	(222)	0
Rhenium	Re	75	186.2	186.22	....
Rhodium	Rh	45	102.905	102.91	3
Rubidium	Rb	37	85.47	85.48	1
Ruthenium	Ru	44	101.07	101.1	3, 4, 6, 8
Samarium	Sm	62	150.35	150.35	2, 3
Scandium	Sc	21	44.956	44.96	3
Selenium	Se	34	78.96	78.96	2, 4, 6
Silicon	Si	14	28.086	28.09	4
Silver, argentum	Ag	47	107.868[1]	107.873	1
Sodium, natrium	Na	11	22.9898	22.991	1
Strontium	Sr	38	87.62	87.63	2
Sulfur	S	16	32.064	32.066*	2, 4, 6
Tantalum	Ta	73	180.948	180.95	5
Technetium	Tc	43	....	(97)	6, 7
Tellurium	Te	52	127.60	127.61	2, 4, 6
Terbium	Tb	65	158.924	158.93	3
Thallium	Tl	81	204.37	204.39	1, 3
Thorium	Th	90	232.038	(232)	4
Thulium	Tm	69	168.934	168.94	3
Tin, stannum	Sn	50	118.69	118.70	2, 4
Titanium	Ti	22	47.90	47.90	3, 4
Tungsten (wolfram)	W	74	183.85	183.86	6
Uranium	U	92	238.03	238.07	4, 6
Vanadium	V	23	50.942	50.95	3, 5
Xenon	Xe	54	131.30	131.30	0
Ytterbium	Yb	70	173.04	173.04	2, 3
Yttrium	Y	39	88.905	88.91	3
Zinc	Zn	30	65.37	65.38	2
Zirconium	Zr	40	91.22	91.22	4

* Because of natural variations in the relative abundances of the isotopes of sulfur the atomic weight of this element has a range of ±0.003.

** The 1959 atomic weights are based on O = 16.000 whereas those of 1966 are based on the isotope C^{12}.

1., ±0.002; 2., ±0.001; 3., ±0.001. From Handbook of chemistry and physics, ed. 50, Weast, R. C., editor, 1969. Used by permission of CRC Press, Inc.

Transmission—optical density table

%T	OD(A)	%T	OD(A)	%T	OD(A)	%T	OD(A)
1.0	2.000	26.0	.585	51.0	.292	76.0	.119
1.5	1.824	26.5	.577	51.5	.288	76.5	.116
2.0	1.699	27.0	.569	52.0	.284	77.0	.114
2.5	1.602	27.5	.561	52.5	.280	77.5	.111
3.0	1.523	28.0	.553	53.0	.276	78.0	.108
3.5	1.456	28.5	.545	53.5	.272	78.5	.105
4.0	1.398	29.0	.538	54.0	.268	79.0	.102
4.5	1.347	29.5	.530	54.5	.264	79.5	.100
5.0	1.301	30.0	.523	55.0	.260	80.0	.097
5.5	1.260	30.5	.516	55.5	.256	80.5	.094
6.0	1.222	31.0	.509	56.0	.252	81.0	.092
6.5	1.187	31.5	.502	56.5	.248	81.5	.089
7.0	1.155	32.0	.495	57.0	.244	82.0	.086
7.5	1.126	32.5	.488	57.5	.240	82.5	.084
8.0	1.097	33.0	.482	58.0	.237	83.0	.081
8.5	1.071	33.5	.475	58.5	.233	83.5	.078
9.0	1.046	34.0	.469	59.0	.229	84.0	.076
9.5	1.022	34.5	.462	59.5	.226	84.5	.073
10.0	1.000	35.0	.456	60.0	.222	85.0	.071
10.5	.979	35.5	.450	60.5	.218	85.5	.068
11.0	.959	36.0	.444	61.0	.215	86.0	.066
11.5	.939	36.5	.438	61.5	.211	86.5	.063
12.0	.921	37.0	.432	62.0	.208	87.0	.061
12.5	.903	37.5	.426	62.5	.204	87.5	.058
13.0	.886	38.0	.420	63.0	.201	88.0	.056
13.5	.870	38.5	.414	63.5	.197	88.5	.053
14.0	.854	39.0	.409	64.0	.194	89.0	.051
14.5	.838	39.5	.403	64.5	.191	89.5	.048
15.0	.824	40.0	.398	65.0	.187	90.0	.046
15.5	.810	40.5	.392	65.5	.184	90.5	.043
16.0	.796	41.0	.387	66.0	.181	91.0	.041
16.5	.782	41.5	.382	66.5	.177	91.5	.039
17.0	.770	42.0	.377	67.0	.174	92.0	.036
17.5	.757	42.5	.372	67.5	.171	92.5	.034
18.0	.745	43.0	.367	68.0	.168	93.0	.032
18.5	.733	43.5	.362	68.5	.164	93.5	.029
19.0	.721	44.0	.357	69.0	.161	94.0	.027
19.5	.710	44.5	.352	69.5	.158	94.5	.025
20.0	.699	45.0	.347	70.0	.155	95.0	.022
20.5	.688	45.5	.342	70.5	.152	95.5	.020
21.0	.678	46.0	.337	71.0	.149	96.0	.018
21.5	.668	46.5	.332	71.5	.146	96.5	.016
22.0	.658	47.0	.328	72.0	.143	97.0	.013
22.5	.648	47.5	.323	72.5	.140	97.5	.011
23.0	.638	48.0	.319	73.0	.137	98.0	.009
23.5	.629	48.5	.314	73.5	.134	98.5	.007
24.0	.620	49.0	.310	74.0	.131	99.0	.004
24.5	.611	49.5	.305	74.5	.128	99.5	.002
25.0	.602	50.0	.301	75.0	.125	100.0	.000
25.5	.594	50.5	.297	75.5	.122		

From Hycel PMS sugar determinations, Houston, Tex., Hycel, Inc.

Nomogram for the determination of body surface area

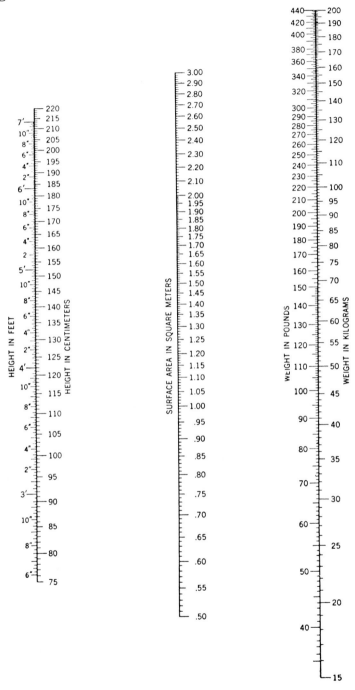

Reprinted, by permission from The New England Journal of Medicine **185**:337, 1921.

Formulas presented in this book

Conversion factors (chapter 3)

To correct when the drug being used as a standard is different from the one being measured

$$\text{Conversion factor} = \frac{\text{mol wt of drug being measured}}{\text{mol wt of drug used as the standard}}$$

To correct for variations in procedure quantities

$$\frac{\text{What should have been used or done}}{\text{What was used or done}} \times \text{Answer}$$

Temperature conversions (chapter 5)

To convert °C to °K

$$°K = °C + 273$$

To convert °K to °C

$$°C = °K - 273$$

To convert °C to °F

$$°F = (°C \times {}^9/_5) + 32$$
$$°F = (°C \times 1.8) + 32$$
$$°F = [(°C + 40) \times {}^9/_5] - 40$$
$$°F = [(°C + 40) \times 1.8] - 40$$

To convert °F to °C

$$°C = (°F - 32) \times {}^5/_9$$
$$°C = (°F - 32) \times 0.556$$
$$°C = [(°F + 40) \times {}^5/_9] - 40$$
$$°C = [(°F + 40) \times 0.556] - 40$$

To convert °C to °F or °F to °C

$$\frac{°C}{°F - 32} = \frac{5}{9}$$
$$9C = 5(F - 32)$$
$$9C = 5F - 160$$

Solutions (chapter 6)

Percent

To find the amount of solute to make a given volume of solution

$$\frac{\text{Percent} \times \text{Desired volume}}{100} = \text{gm (or ml) of solute to be diluted up to the desired volume}$$

To find the percent of a solution when the amount of solute and total volume of solution are known

$$\frac{\text{gm (or ml) of solute} \times 100}{\text{Volume of solution}} = \text{Percent}$$

When changing concentration or performing titration procedures

$$V_1 \times C_1 = V_2 \times C_2$$

When mixing two or more solutions together

$$(V_1 \times C_1) + (V_2 \times C_2) + (V_3 \times C_3) + \ldots = V_F \times C_F$$

Molarity

$$\text{mol wt} \times \text{M} = \text{gm/l}$$

$$\text{M} = \frac{\text{gm/l}}{\text{mol wt}}$$

$$\text{mmoles/l} = \frac{\text{mg/l}}{\text{mol wt}}$$

Osmolarity

Osmolarity (osmoles/l) = M × Particles/Molecule resulting from ionization

Milliosmolarity (mOsmoles/l) = mmoles/l × Particles/Molecule resulting from ionization

$$\text{osmoles/l} = \frac{\Delta \text{ temperature}}{1.86}$$

$$\text{mOsmoles/l} = \frac{\Delta \text{ temperature}}{0.00186}$$

Normality

$$\text{eq wt} \times \text{N} = \text{gm/l}$$

$$\text{N} = \frac{\text{gm/l}}{\text{eq wt}}$$

Specific gravity

$$\text{sp gr} \times \text{\% purity (as decimal)} = \text{gm specific solute/ml}$$

$$\text{sp gr} = \frac{\text{Weight of solid or liquid}}{\text{Weight of equal volume of } H_2O \text{ at } 4°C}$$

Concentration relationships

To convert $\%^{w/v}$ to molarity *or* molarity to $\%^{w/v}$

$$\text{M} = \frac{\%^{w/v} \times 10}{\text{mol wt}}$$

To convert $\%^{w/v}$ to normality *or* normality to $\%^{w/v}$

$$\text{N} = \frac{\%^{w/v} \times 10}{\text{eq wt}}$$

To convert mg/dl to mEq/l *or* mEq/l to mg/dl

$$\text{mEq/l} = \frac{\text{mg/dl} \times 10}{\text{eq wt}}$$

To convert molarity to normality

$$\text{N} = \text{M} \times \text{Valence}$$

To convert normality to molarity

$$M = \frac{N}{\text{Valence}}$$

To convert vol% CO_2 to mmoles/l CO_2

$$\text{mmoles/l} = \text{vol\%} \times 0.45$$

To convert mmoles/l CO_2 to vol% CO_2

$$\text{vol\%} = \text{mmoles/l} \times 2.226$$

Ionic concentration and pH (chapter 7)

pH—pOH

$$[H^+] \times [OH^-] = 1 \times 10^{-14}$$

$$pH + pOH = 14$$

$$N \times \text{\% ionization} = [H^+]$$

$$pH = \log \frac{1}{[H^+]}$$

$$pH = -\log [H^+]$$

$$pH = b - \log a \text{ (using } [H^+] \text{ expressed in scientific notation)}$$

$$pOH = \log \frac{1}{[OH^-]}$$

$$pOH = -\log [OH^-]$$

$$pOH = b - \log a \text{ (using } [OH^-] \text{ expressed in scientific notation)}$$

Henderson-Hasselbalch equation

$$pH = pK + \log \frac{[\text{salt}]}{[\text{acid}]}$$

$$pH = pK + \log \frac{[HCO_3^-]}{[CO_2]}$$

$$pH = pK + \log \frac{\text{Total } CO_2 - a \times P_{CO_2}}{a \times P_{CO_2}}$$

$$P_{CO_2} \text{ (mmoles Hg)} = \frac{\text{Total } CO_2 \text{ (mmoles/l)}}{0.03 \, [\text{antilog(pH} - 6.1) + 1]}$$

$$\text{Total } CO_2 \text{ (mmoles/l)} = 0.03 \, P_{CO_2} \, [\text{antilog(pH} - 6.1) + 1]$$

Dilutions (chapter 8)

Original concentration $\times$ Dilution 1 $\times$ Dilution 2 $\times$ Dilution 3 $\times$ . . . = Final concentration

Colorimetry (chapter 9)

To calculate the concentration of an unknown that follows Beer's law

$$C_u = \frac{A_u}{A_s} \times C_s$$

Relationship between absorbance and percent transmittance

$$A = \log \frac{1}{T}$$

$$A = -\log T$$

$$A = 2 - \log \%T$$

Relationship between absorbance, molar absorptivity, and concentration

$$A = \epsilon \times C \times d$$

Standard curves (chapter 10)

To calculate the concentration of a standard for a given test

$$C_s = W_s \times D \times \frac{V_c}{V_t}$$

$$C_s = \text{ml } WS \text{ std} \times \frac{100}{\text{Quantity of sample used}} \times \text{conc } WS/\text{ml}$$

Hematology math (chapter 11)

To calculate a final factor when using diluting pipettes and the counting chamber

$$\text{Dilution factor} \times \text{Depth factor} \times \frac{1}{\text{Area counted}} = \text{Final factor}$$

$$\text{Dilution factor} \times \text{Depth factor} \times \text{Area factor} = \text{Final factor}$$

$$\text{Dilution factor} \times \frac{1}{\text{Volume counted}} = \text{Final factor}$$

$$\text{Dilution factor} \times \text{Volume factor} = \text{Final factor}$$

$$\frac{\text{Dilution factor} \times \text{Depth factor}}{\text{Area counted}} = \text{Final factor}$$

To find the area factor

$$\text{Area factor} = \frac{1}{\text{Area counted}}$$

To find the volume factor

$$\text{Volume factor} = \frac{1}{\text{Volume counted}}$$

$$\text{Volume factor} = \text{Depth factor} \times \text{Area factor}$$

To find the mean corpuscular volume

$$\text{MCV} = \frac{\text{Hct} \times 10}{\text{RBC (in millions)}}$$

To find the mean corpuscular hemoglobin

$$\text{MCH} = \frac{\text{Hb (in grams)} \times 10}{\text{RBC (in millions)}}$$

To find the mean corpuscular hemoglobin concentration

$$\text{MCHC} = \frac{\text{Hb (in grams)} \times 100}{\text{Hct}}$$

To find the concentration for a hemoglobin standard in a given procedure

$$\frac{\text{Conc of std (assay)} \times \text{Dilution factor}}{1000} = \text{gm}\%$$

Enzyme calculations (chapter 12)

To calculate international units per liter

$$IU/l = \frac{\Delta A_{340}/\min \times V_t}{6.22 \times V_s} \times 1000 \times \frac{1}{t}$$

$$IU/l = \frac{\Delta A_{334}/\min \times V_t}{6.0 \times V_s} \times 1000 \times \frac{1}{t}$$

$$IU/l = \frac{\Delta A_{366}/\min \times V_t}{3.3 \times V_s} \times 1000 \times \frac{1}{t}$$

$$IU/l = \mu moles/\min/l$$

To calculate IU/ml

$$IU/ml = \mu moles/\min/ml$$

Calculations based on ϵ and the absorbance

$$IU/l = \frac{A \text{ of sample}}{\epsilon \times d} \times 10^6 \times \frac{1}{t} \times \frac{V_t}{V_s}$$

Calculations based on a standard

$$IU/l = \frac{A \text{ of sample}}{A \text{ of standard}} \times 10^6 \times [\text{Standard}] \times \frac{1}{t} \times \frac{V_t}{V_s}$$

Renal clearance tests (chapter 14)

Creatinine clearance
Uncorrected

$$C = \frac{U}{P} \times V$$

Corrected for body surface

$$C = \frac{U}{P} \times V \times \frac{1.73}{A}$$

Urea clearance
Maximum, uncorrected

$$C = \frac{U}{P} \times V$$

Maximum, corrected for body surface

$$C = \frac{U}{P} \times V \times \frac{1.73}{A}$$

Maximum, corrected for body surface and reported in percent of normal

$$C = \frac{U}{P} \times V \times \frac{1.73}{A} \times \frac{100}{75}$$

Standard, uncorrected

$$C = \frac{U}{P} \times \sqrt{V}$$

Standard, corrected for body surface

$$C = \frac{U}{P} \times \sqrt{V} \times \frac{1.73}{A}$$

Standard, corrected for body surface and reported in percent of normal

$$C = \frac{U}{P} \times \sqrt{V} \times \frac{1.73}{A} \times \frac{100}{54}$$

Body surface in square meters

$$\log A = (0.425 \times \log W) + (0.725 \times \log H) - 2.144$$

Quality control (chapter 15)

Variance

$$s^2 = \frac{\Sigma(X-\overline{X})^2}{n-1}$$

Standard deviation

$$s = \sqrt{s^2}$$

$$s = \sqrt{\frac{\Sigma(X-\overline{X})^2}{n-1}}$$

% Coefficient of variation

$$\%CV = \frac{s}{\overline{X}} \times 100$$

Answers to practice problems

Chapter 1

1. +97
2. −4
3. −26
4. +13
5. −1
6. +1
7. −13
8. +3
9. −11
10. +16
11. +17
12. −21
13. +7
14. −13
15. +13
16. −7
17. +48
18. −14
19. −40
20. +39
21. +20
22. −20
23. −20
24. +20
25. +22
26. −0.5
27. −5
28. +0.5
29. +5
30. −5
31. −5
32. +5
33. $\frac{1}{10}$
34. 8
35. $\frac{1}{1.16}$; 0.862
36. −23
37. +115.5
38. −5.75
39. +380
40. $\frac{1}{16}$
41. $\frac{21}{12}$; $\frac{7}{4}$; $1\frac{3}{4}$
42. $\frac{17}{24}$

43. $\frac{1}{27}$
44. 1
45. $\frac{22}{40}$; $\frac{11}{20}$
46. $\frac{9}{3}$; 3
47. $\frac{68}{24}$; $\frac{34}{12}$; $\frac{17}{6}$; $2\frac{5}{6}$
48. $\frac{138}{30}$; $\frac{69}{15}$; $\frac{23}{5}$; $4\frac{3}{5}$
49. $\frac{2}{9}$
50. $\frac{6}{10}$; $\frac{3}{5}$
51. $-\frac{61}{15}$; $-4\frac{1}{15}$
52. 10,000,000
53. 100
54. 0.0001
55. 7776
56. $\frac{1}{8}$; 0.125
57. 10,000
58. 0.000001
59. 1,010,000
60. a^8
61. $b^3 \times c^2$
62. 713
63. a^3
64. a^5
65. 1100
66. 0.010001
67. 10,077,696
68. 25
69. 10,000
70. 0.000001
71. 9,529,569
72. 10:8; 10/8; 10 to 8; 1.25
73. a. 2:8
    b. 8:2
    c. 2:10
    d. 10:2
    e. 8:10
    f. 10:8

74. $X = 4$; $\frac{1}{2} = \frac{4}{8}$
75. $X = 2.5$; $\frac{2.5}{10} = \frac{1}{4}$
76. $X = 4$; $\frac{2}{4} = \frac{3}{6}$
77. $X = 25$; $\frac{4}{20} = \frac{5}{25}$
78. 4 gm
79. 50 ml
80. 6 gm
81. a. 5.0×10^6
    b. 1.42×10^5
    c. 5.9×10^4
    d. 1.72×10^{-5}
    e. 1.11×10^{-3}
    f. 2.91×10^{-9}
82. a. 1.15038×10^{12}
    b. 3.952×10^9
    c. 6.25×10^{-7}
    d. 2.2×10^1
    e. 4.58×10^{-3}

Chapter 2

1. 3.721
2. 0.721
3. $\overline{3}$.721; 7.721 − 10
4. $\overline{1}$.721; 9.721 − 10
5. 1.721
6. 2.1402
7. $\overline{2}$.9968; 8.9968 − 10
8. 1.3370
9. 0.7055
10. $\overline{5}$.8997; 5.8997 − 10
11. 2,099,907
12. 0.296
13. 0.0153
14. 4460

15. 0.000107
16. 89.39
17. 7.435
18. 0.00524
19. 5240
20. 5.244
21. 0.02096
22. 109.4
23. 180.8
24. 32412
25. 0.00005767
   log 624 = 2.7952 = 12.7952 − 10
   antilog $\overline{5}$.7609 = 0.00005767

Chapter 3

1. 1.29
2. 0.39
3. Factor = 1.65; 495 mg/dl
4. Factor = 0.78; 390 mg/dl

5. Factor = 0.95; 47.5 mg/dl
6. 40
7. 300 mg/dl
8. 500 mg/dl

Chapter 4

1. 95.45 kg
2. 177.8 cm; 1.778 m
3. a. 6 dg
   b. 0.15 cg
   c. 60,000,000 ng
   d. 0.05 kg
   e. 360,000 mg
4. a. 1 ml
   b. 5000 ml
   c. 60,000 ml

5. 0.0006 cm
6. d
7. 90,909 gm
8. 0.5644 oz
9. 2.34 gallons
10. a. 0.006 dl
    b. 3000 cg
    c. 2.74 m
    d. 0.94 lb
    e. 9.472 l

Chapter 5

1. 77°F
2. −4°F
3. 500°F

4. 65.56°C
5. −28.89°C
6. 204.44°C

Chapter 6

1. 60 ml of 10% ↑ 100 ml
2. 27 ml of 10% ↑ 30 ml
3. 600 ml HCl ↑ 2000 ml
4. 10%
5. 1 gm
6. None; a stronger solution cannot be made from a weaker one.
7. 125 ml
8. 600 gm ↑ 2000 ml
9. 5.25 ml
10. 8.3%
11. 250 ml
12. 22.05 gm Na_2SO_4 ↑ 500 ml
13. 393.24 gm $CaCl_2 \cdot 10H_2O$ ↑ 3000 ml
14. 180 gm
15. 5.13м

16. 4.1M
17. 0.375M
18. 250 ml
19. 1.2M
20. 40
21. 11.1 gm/l
22. 48 gm
23. None; read the question.
24. 600 ml
25. 10 osmoles/l
26. 50 mOsmoles/l
27. 246.2 mOsmoles/l
28. 381.7 mOsmoles/l
29. $-0.37°C$
30. a. 344.6 mOsmoles/l NaCl
    b. 0.172M
31. 98.1 gm H_3PO_4 ↑ 500 ml
32. 27.78 gm $CaCl_2$ ↑ 100 ml
33. 1000 ml H_2O
34. 2.5N
35. 6 ml
36. 80 ml
37. 12.17 gm ↑ 2000 ml
38. 8N
39. 117 gm
40. 294 gm H_3PO_4 ↑ 3 l
41. 20 mEq
42. 5.21 gm ↑ 200 ml
43. 0.1N
44. 1.167 gm ↑ 250 ml
45. 180 ml
46. 87.4 gm $CaCl_2 \cdot 10H_2O$ ↑ 300 ml
47. 220.5 gm H_2SO_4 ↑ 1500 ml
48. 14 lb; $44.80
49. 10N
50. 1.54N
51. 83.33 ml
52. 6N
53. 666.7 ml 3N + 1333.3 ml 6N
54. 4 ml 10N ↑ 100 ml

55. 28.17N
56. 1.41N
57. 31.5 gm
58. 45.22 gm
59. 87.85 ml H_2SO_4 ↑ 400 ml
60. 6%$^{v/v}$; 10.70%$^{w/v}$
61. 380.28 ml HNO_3 ↑ 1000 ml
62. a. 12.5%$^{v/v}$
    b. 5.65%$^{w/v}$
    c. 1.55M
    d. 1.55N
63. a. 12.38M; 12.38N
    b. 18.21M; 36.42N
    c. 15.8M; 15.8N
64. 303.58 ml conc + 500 ml 10% ↑ 1000 ml
65. 56.91%$^{v/v}$
66. 100.62 ml H_2O
67. 83.13 mEq/l Cl
68. 526.5 mg/dl NaCl
69. 40 ml
70. 3M H_2SO_4 *is* 6N
71. Impossible
72. 10.95%$^{w/v}$
73. 3.17N; 3.17M
74. a. 5 mEq/l
    b. 119.66 mEq/l
    c. 3.58 mEq/l
75. 0.145N
76. a. 322 mg/dl
    b. 10 mg/dl
    c. 19.5 mg/dl
77. 48 ml
78. 241.9 ml
79. 7.5N
80. 10.71%$^{w/v}$
81. 100 ml
82. 2.5M
83. 9N
84. 0.145M; 0.145N

Chapter 7

1. b
2. 0.48 gm H^+/l
3. 8.0
4. 1×10^{-8}
5. 5.0
7. 3.162×10^{-3} or 0.003162 moles/l HCl; 0.0006324 moles HCl/200 ml
8. 5.5086
9. 3.2676
10. 1.585×10^{-8}
11. 1.096×10^{-3}
12. 0.087 moles/l acid = 0.087 × 60 = 5.22 gm/l acid
    0.113 moles/l salt = 0.113 × 82 = 9.266 gm/l salt

6. a. 0.021
    b. 0.476×10^{-12}
    c. 1.6778
    d. 12.3222

Chapter 8

1. 2:32 dilution; 2:30 ratio
2. a. 1:9
   b. 3:24
   c. 6:3
   d. 40:10
3. a. 1/10
   b. 1/9
   c. 1/1.5
   d. 1/1.25
4. 3.5/4; 0.875/l; 1/1.14
5. $\dfrac{1}{10} \times \dfrac{1}{10} \times \dfrac{1}{100} = \dfrac{1}{10,000}$
6. a. Place 1 ml of 10N NaOH in one tube and dilute up to a total volume of 10 ml.
   b. Place 1 ml from this tube into another tube and dilute up to a total volume of 5 ml.
   c. Place 3 ml from the preceding tube into another tube and dilute up to a total volume of 15 ml.
7. 15 ml
8. $\dfrac{1}{25}$N or 0.04N
9. 0.06 ml
10. 0.5 mg/ml
11. Tube 4 = 1:1296
    Tube 8 = 1:1,679,616
12. Volume = 50 ml

    Concentration = $\dfrac{20}{50}$% or 0.4%
13. 1/250 dilution
14. $\dfrac{40}{1000} \times \dfrac{X}{50} = \dfrac{1}{300}$

    $X = 4.17$

    4.17 oz stock solution diluted up to 50 oz would give 50 oz of a 1:300 solution.
15. $\dfrac{1}{100} \times \dfrac{X}{8} = \dfrac{1}{500}$

    $X = 1.6$

    1.6 oz of stock solution diluted up to 8 oz would give 8 oz of a 1:500 solution.

Chapter 9

1. $C_u = \dfrac{L_s}{L_u} \times C_s$

2. $C_u = \dfrac{A_u}{A_s} \times C_s$

3. *$A = \log \dfrac{1}{T}$

    $A = \log 1 - \log T$
    $A = 0 - \log T$
    *$A = -\log T$

    $A = -\log \dfrac{\%T}{100}$

    $A = -(\log \%T - \log 100)$
    $A = -(\log \%T - 2)$
    $A = -\log \%T + 2$
    *$A = 2 - \log \%T$

4. Absorbance is a measure of the amount of light stopped by a solution.

---

*One of three main formulas.

5. Transmission is a mathematical comparison of the amount of light emerging from a solution to the amount of light entering the solution.
6. Transmittance value is the comparison of the transmission of the unknown solution to the transmission of the blank solution.
7. %T is the transmittance value times 100.

Chapter 10

1. 47.14 gm/dl
2. 0.025 ml *SS* ↑ 50 ml
3. 0.2 mg/ml
4. 1 ml *SS* ↑ 10 ml
5. 10 mg%
6. a. 350 mg/dl
   b. 0.3 ml
   c. 0.35 mg/ml
   d. 0.7 ml *SS* ↑ 10 ml
   e. $\left(0.3 \times \dfrac{100}{0.03}\right) 0.35 = 350$

$\left(0.2 \times \dfrac{100}{0.03}\right) 0.35 = 233.3$

$\left(0.1 \times \dfrac{100}{0.03}\right) 0.35 = 116.7$

7. 600 mEq/l
   2130 mg/dl
8. 0.2 mEq
9. 40 mEq/l
   56 mg/dl
10. 10 mg/dl

Chapter 11

1. $\dfrac{1}{20}$

2. $\dfrac{1}{50}$

3. $\dfrac{1}{125}$

4. $\dfrac{1}{100}$

5. a. 33.3
   b. 10
   c. 0.1
   d. 1
   e. 33.3
6. A. 3 mm
   B. 1 mm
11. 10.9 gm%

C. 0.25 mm
D. 0.2 mm
E. 0.05 mm
F. 1 mm²
G. 0.0625 mm²
H. 0.04 mm²
I. 0.0025 mm²
7. a. 100
   b. 0.111
   c. 111.1
8. 5666 platelets/mm³
9. 20,000 WBC/mm³
   30,000 NRBC/mm³
10. a. 88.2 μm³
    b. 30.4 $\mu\mu$gm
    c. 34.4%

Sample	Diluent (ml)	Standard (ml)	Value (gm%)
1.	0	6.0	10.9
2.	1.5	4.5	8.2
3.	3.0	3.0	5.5
4.	4.5	1.5	2.7
5.	6.0	0	0

This is one method.

Chapter 12

1. 3.53
2. 5.4
3. 16.7
4. 0.482

Chapter 13

1. 100 ml
2. 100 ml
3. 1000 ml
4. Free = 24°; 24 mEq/l
   Combined = 16°; 16 mEq/l
   Total = 40°; 40 mEq/l

5. 45°
6. 41 mEq/l
7. Free = 6.8°; 6.8 mEq/l
   Combined = 12.2°; 12.2 mEq/l
   Total = 19°; 19 mEq/l

Chapter 14

1. a. 2.19 m²
   b. 0.79
2. 41.7 ml/min
3. 62.5 ml/min; 83.3% of normal

4. a. 1.68 m²
   b. 1.03
   c. 11.18 ml/min (uncorrected)
   d. 11.52 (corrected)
   e. 21.3% of normal (corrected)
   f. 20.7% of normal (uncorrected)

References

Annino, J. S.: Clinical chemistry, principles and practices, ed 3, Boston, 1964, Little, Brown and Company.

Davidsohn, I., and Henry, J.: Todd-Sanford clinical diagnosis by laboratory methods, ed. 15, Philadelphia, 1974, W. B. Saunders Company.

Dybkaer, R., and Jørgensen, K.: Quantities and units in clinical chemistry; including Recommendation 1966 of the Commission on Clinical Chemistry of the International Union of Pure and Applied Chemistry and of the International Federation for Clinical Chemistry, Copenhagen, 1967, Munksgaard, International Booksellers & Publishers Ltd., and Baltimore, 1967, The Williams & Wilkins Company.

Henry, R. J., Cannon, D. C., and Winkelman, J. W.: Clinical chemistry-principles and technics, ed. 2, New York, 1974, Harper & Row, Publishers.

Lynch, M. J., Raphael, S. S., Mellor, L. D., Spare, P. D., and Inwood, M. J. H.: Medical laboratory technology and clinical pathology, Philadelphia, 1969, W. B. Saunders Company.

Martinek, R. G.: Practical mathematics for the medical technologist, J. Am. Med. Tech. **34:**117-146, 1972.

Mattenheimer, H.: The theory of enzyme tests, New York and San Francisco, Boehringer Mannheim Corporation.

Oser, B. L., editor: Hawk's physiological chemistry, ed. 14, New York, 1965, McGraw-Hill Book Company.

Perkin-Elmer: Model 54 spectrophotometer systems enzyme workshop manual, Colman Instruments Division.

Robinson, J. W.: Undergraduate instrumental analaysis, ed 2, New York, 1973, Marcel Dekker, Inc.

Routh, J. I.: Mathematical preparation for laboratory technicians, Philadelphia, 1971, W. B. Saunders Company.

Tietz, N. W., editor: Fundamentals of clinical chemistry, Philadelphia, 1970, W. B. Saunders Company.

White, W. L., Erickson, M. M., and Stevens, S. C.: Chemistry for medical technologists, ed. 3, St. Louis, 1970, The C. V. Mosby Company.

Willard, H. H., Merritt, L. L., Jr., and Dean, J. A.: Instrumental methods of analysis, ed. 4, New York, 1965, D. Van Nostrand Company.

Index